KT-498-706

Antenatal Education:
A Dynamic Approach

Mary Nolan
Antenatal Teacher/Tutor
The National Childbirth Trust

Baillière Tindall

LONDON   EDINBURGH   NEW YORK   PHILADELPHIA   SYDNEY   TORONTO   1998

12180

D0541928

Antenatal Education

The Library
Education Centre, Royal Surrey County Hospital
Egerton Road, Guildford, Surrey GU2 7XX
Tel: 01483 464137

Class no: WQ 150 *Computer no:* H9904114

Baillière Tindall
An imprint of Harcourt Brace and Company Limited

Baillière Tindall, 24–28 Oval Road, London NW1 7DX

The Curtis Center, Independence Square West, Philadelphia, PA 19106-3399, USA

Harcourt Brace & Company, 55 Horner Avenue, Toronto, Ontario, M8Z 4X6, Canada

Harcourt Brace & Company – Australia, 30–52 Smidmore Street, Marrickville, NSW 2204, Australia

Harcourt Brace & Company – Japan, Ichibancho Central Building, 22–1 Ichibancho, Chiyoda-ku, Tokyo 102, Japan

© 1998 Harcourt Brace and Company Limited

This book is printed on acid-free paper

All rights reserved. No part of this publication may be reproduced,
stored in a retrieval system or transmitted, in any form or by any other
means, electronic, mechanical, photocopying or otherwise, without the prior
permission of Baillière Tindall, 24–28 Oval Road, London NW1 7DX

A catalogue record for this book is available from the British Library

ISBN 0-7020-2279-9

Typeset by Phoenix Photosetting, Chatham, Kent
Printed and bound in Great Britain by Bell and Bain Ltd, Glasgow

Contents

Introduction

I hope that this book conveys my passionate enthusiasm for and commitment to childbirth education. Only 40 years ago, the idea of classes to help women prepare for having a baby and becoming a mother was novel. Now, it is mainstream. Not only do almost 50% of women expecting their first babies attend some kind of antenatal classes, but so do many of their partners, friends and family members. The problem for childbirth educators today, as for any group of people who were once revolutionaries and then find themselves part of the 'establishment', is that the impetus that once drove them forward may become sluggish. To re-energize educators is the aim of this book because, when expectant parents come away from antenatal classes feeling that they have learned very little, that the class was irrelevant or boring, a precious opportunity has been lost.

It is quite evident that, in the highly developed world, preparation for birth and parenting is crucial – crucial because we are so far removed, both physically and emotionally, from birth. Our understanding of how women feel about giving birth and how they feel when they have given birth, and of the immensely powerful resources women have for coping in labour, is sadly limited. Childbirth educators have the chance to put women back in touch with their instincts, and to increase the confidence of all parents-to-be that they really do know how to look after their children and do not need to rely on 'experts'.

In this book, I have described the person who provides learning opportunities for pregnant women and their partners as a Childbirth Educator. Perhaps in the UK it is more usual to hear the term 'antenatal teacher' or 'parentcraft teacher'. 'Teacher' is, however, a noun fraught with connotations of school and pedagogy, and what this book is trying hard to say is that antenatal education is about educating *adults* and that, with a little skilled assistance, adults can educate themselves.

At the moment, most childbirth educators work in the antenatal period only as the term 'antenatal teacher' implies. I've chosen the term '*childbirth* educator' because I think we need to broaden our concept of childbirth education and extend the availability of education to parents from the antenatal period into the first weeks and months of their babies' lives. Labour and giving birth are climactic events in the life of a woman and her family; but they are short-lived (although long remembered). Parenting, as we all know, is for ever and the support that a woman receives from her childbirth educator before the birth should not, in an ideal situation, come to an end once the birth has taken place – when she most needs it.

This book is about working with *groups* of expectant parents and their supporters, but the educational concepts that underpin it can be applied to every situation in which health professionals and childbirth educators have the opportunity to educate. Such occasions are multiple and embrace all those occasions when a woman on her own or with her partner meets a health professional or childbirth educator with the skills to enable her to learn more about the business of becoming a parent.

Acknowledgements

I am indebted to a huge number of people in the writing of this book. In particular, I would like to mention Elisabeth Buggins, Helen Davies, Chris Carson, Lorna Brown, Lorna Hartwell, Mary Smale and all the students whom I have trained to be childbirth educators. To the teachers, tutors, counsellors and members of The National Childbirth Trust, I owe more than I can ever express. My gratitude to each and every parent whom I have taught during my career as a childbirth educator goes without saying.

Mary Nolan

Evidence-based Practice in Antenatal Education

A BRIEF HISTORY OF ANTENATAL EDUCATION

Antenatal education has a long history. It is a history that has little to do with the formal provision of classes. Rather it is a history of the ways in which women have cared for and communicated with each other down the centuries. Just as today, children's earliest information about babies and how they come into the world is generally gained from their mothers, so knowledge of childbirth and childrearing has traditionally been passed from one generation of women to the next through an oral tradition.

In most parts of the world, it is unheard of for men to be present while women are giving birth. Women have guarded the privacy, some might say sanctity, of birth by keeping the business of birthing to themselves. In traditional cultures, a young girl learns about pregnancy through her daily proximity to pregnant women of the tribe or village community and by attending births in the capacity of either witness or supporter. In such communities, women are assisted during labour by other women – their mother, their sister, their friends or the village 'wise woman' (Priya, 1992). Women learn how to give birth by watching other women giving birth; they also learn that birth may be a joyful event or it may be a tragic one, that some babies live and some die. The anthropologist Margaret Mead (1943) described how even very small children:

> watched miscarriage and peeped under the arms of the old women who were washing and commenting upon the undeveloped foetus. (p 110)

For thousands of years, it was the 'women's network' which, in all parts of the world, kept women informed about labour and birth. Each small community shared an understanding of what having a baby was really like. Whilst women supported each other during labour, knowledge of the process of birth, of what helped and what hindered it, of how women react during labour and how new-born babies look and behave, was part of every woman's understanding of herself and her role. Acquiring this knowledge was part of the socialization of young girls.

This situation began gradually to change in the mid-eighteenth century when the Industrial Revolution created a middle class of successful entrepreneurs who could afford to build large houses, employ servants and live lives that were separate from their neighbours'. Factories were built and the centre of employment shifted away from the countryside and its traditional small communities and into the towns. The wives of factory owners and industrialists did not work as their mothers and grandmothers had done:

> In pre-industrial Britain, then, a woman's role in adult life was always the role of productive worker ... As well as economic changes, industrialization profoundly altered women's family roles ... The concept of private, home-centred family life is now a primary social value, while it had hardly begun to be so in the seventeenth century. (Oakley, 1976, pp 30–31)

Home-centred family life did not mean that women necessarily participated in childcare. The babies of middle-class women were often wet-nursed and their children cared for by servants and later tutors and governesses. Women no longer attended each other's births. It was increasingly fashionable to hire an accoucheur for labour, a male doctor who brought with him instruments such as forceps which were supposed to make birth easier, safer and more civilized. Middle-class women thus became separated from the women's network and their understanding of their bodies and their confidence in birth were eroded as their everyday involvement in the pregnancies and births of other women was reduced.

Working-class women may have lived physically closer to each other in the new manufacturing towns than they had done when their families tilled the land in the pre-industrial era. However, they no longer worked in and around their homes but in factories which removed them from the intimacies of family life. Giving birth at home, supported by family members and neighbours, became far less attractive to women than it had been. Those who would have supported them in labour could not leave the looms and spinning jennies to be with them as they could once have left the fields or the spinning wheel; nor was a Victorian slum a suitable environment in which to give birth. By the late nineteenth and early twentieth centuries, working-class women were increasingly choosing to give birth in the public hospitals despite the ravages of puerperal fever. Being in hospital allowed them access to the doctors whom they knew attended the births of wealthier women. The medical profession held out the promise of less painful and safer childbearing. Queen Victoria delivered her last two babies under chloroform, and inhalational analgesia became increasingly popular despite its evident risks. Working-class women, whose poor health put them at increased likelihood of childbed complications, were attracted into the hospitals by the lure of pain relief to help them cope with what might be long, obstructed or otherwise difficult labours. Hospitalization provided them with a respite from the demands of their working lives and the care of large numbers of children who were no longer seen as belonging to a community that shared the burden of their upbringing, but as the sole responsibility of their parents. Many women found themselves ground down by ignorance, fear, relentless childbearing and lack of support:

> Can we wonder that so many women take drugs, hoping to get rid of the expected child, when they know so little regarding their own bodies, and have to work so hard to keep or help to keep the children they have already got? (Llewelyn Davies 1915; c.f. Dallas, 1989)

Victorian women were, of course, aware that they now approached childbirth with little of the understanding or wisdom that had benefited their ancestors. There was a great thirst for the kind of knowledge that they had once acquired as a part of growing up. Magazines such as 'Enquire Within About Everything', which answered women's questions about sex and reproduction, found a ready market. 'Enquire Within About Everything' was written by men, mainly doctors and clergymen, and was, not surprisingly, sometimes patronizing and coy, but it did provide information to women who were approaching marriage or childbearing in a state of fear and ignorance.

The influence of the Eugenics movement, which aimed to improve the population through policies to control breeding, encouraged governments of the late nineteenth and early twentieth centuries to turn an eye towards the quality of the nation's manhood which was found to be unacceptably low. In an effort to address this, women – especially poor women – were targeted with health information to inspire them to take better care of themselves during pregnancy and of their infants when they were born. The medical profession's increasingly wide remit for the care and control of childbearing women was reflected in the literature written by doctors at this time:

> The writers adopt a(n) ... authoritarian style, laying down 'laws of health', 'commandments' and 'rules' rather than offering 'hints' and 'advice'. The difference in vocabulary reflects a more fundamental change in approach: from an emphasis upon self-control to one upon medical control ... a scientific morality where it is the doctor rather than God and nature who is omnipotent. (Graham, 1977, p 21)

Whilst little was done to attack the profound social causes of infant mortality and childhood morbidity for which women were not responsible – poverty, inadequate housing and poor sanitation – public health authorities throughout the UK did move to establish milk depots which provided uncontaminated milk for mothers to give their babies and young children. The house of a child placed on the list to receive free milk would then be visited by a lady sanitary inspector who gave the mother instruction on basic hygiene and infant management:

> By 1906, when the first National Conference on Infantile Mortality was held in London, it had become a general assumption among medical professionals, health care administrators, and policy makers, that the correct education of mothers was an integral part of the struggle to lower infant mortality. (Oakley, 1984, p 42)

Home visiting to educate mothers about the proper care of their families became the key role of the first Health Visitors, a large number of whom in the early years of the century were volunteers. Health Visitors also gave advice to pregnant women and continued to be the main official providers of antenatal education until the 1950s when, with the increase in the number of hospital confinements, antenatal education became a part of the midwife's role.

The increasing demand from government and women themselves for education in the antenatal as well as postnatal period and the medical profession's escalating power over the management of labour combined to generate new ideas about how best to control the pain of labour and how to enable women to cooperate effectively with their medical carers. Medical thinking focused on whether the pain of labour was a physiological function of the contraction of the uterus or a cultural construct based on women's ignorance and fear of the birth process. In Russia, Velvovski considered that the contraction of the uterine muscle was of itself painless and that, if women could be taught how to relax during labour, they would feel no pain. His ideas were taken up by Dick-Read in Britain and by Lamaze in France.

Fernand Lamaze did not subscribe to the theory that contractions were painless, but he did believe that women could be taught how to distract themselves from the pain by concentrating on stimuli other than those coming from the uterus. His ideas owed much to Pavlov's work on conditioned reflexes.

Grantly Dick-Read was very much influenced by his own experience of helping women give birth. Once, when attending a young woman in the East End of London, he was amazed to observe that she delivered her baby with no expressions or signs of discomfort at all. When questioned after the birth, the mother replied that she did not know that labour was *supposed* to hurt. From this, Dick-Read deduced that birth could be painless for women and that it was women's tension that made contractions painful. He devised the model that describes how fear of labour causes the mother to become tense and her tension causes her to feel pain (Fig. 1.1).

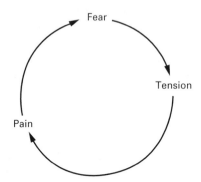

FIG. 1.1   *The Dick-Read model proposes that fear of labour causes the mother to become tense and her tension causes her to feel pain.*

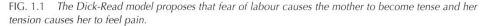

In practice, Dick-Read and Lamaze advocated similar strategies for preparing women for childbirth, although the theory underpinning their approaches was different. Both believed that the pregnant woman should be educated not only because education is valuable on a social level to raise the general standard of knowledge, but also because telling the woman what is going to happen to her reduces her fear; giving her knowledge increases her self-esteem; and helping her understand the birth process enables better communication with her carers.

Dick-Read suggested that women should be taught how to relax all the muscles not associated with the birth process. If the woman could be coached to a sufficiently high standard, her relaxation skills would then enable her to experience childbirth as the painless phenomenon it naturally is.

Lamaze considered that childbirth preparation should include instruction in relaxation based on breathing patterns, which were to be used as a distraction technique. The relaxation skills taught at Lamaze classes demand intense mental concentration in order to be effective and some educators advise that breathing patterns should not be employed until labour is well established or the woman runs the risk of mental exhaustion.

The ideas of Dick-Read and Lamaze were in tune with many women's aspirations, namely to learn more about birth and so have more control over the management of their labours. In France, Lamaze-style prepared childbirth classes became very popular and were endorsed by the Pope, who considered that such education safeguarded the normal reproductive process and encouraged self-control in women. In the UK, Dick-Read's ideas were taken up by an enthusiastic group of women headed by Prunella Briance, who formed the Natural Childbirth Association in 1956 later to become the National Childbirth Trust. The NCT provided antenatal classes run by women whose primary qualification in childbirth education was that they had themselves given birth. The organization was founded on an ethos of support for women who were embarking on motherhood from women who were experienced mothers.

The interplay, sometimes creative and sometimes hostile, between antenatal classes offered by midwives and those provided by the NCT fostered the development of antenatal education. The women who came to classes, whether at the hospital or in the home of an NCT teacher, were the descendants of those middle-class women who, in the late eighteenth century, had begun to find themselves cut off from traditional sources of wisdom about birth and early parenting. From the 1950s onwards, antenatal education was organized to accommodate the learning styles of women who had the time to set aside for antenatal classes and the confidence to articulate their needs and negotiate with hospital staff. These women were comfortable in a situation where they were given information and expected to socialize and engage in discussion with women they had not met before. Those for whom access to the women's network continued – women living in small, often rural, communities or in extended families – did not come to antenatal classes. Nor did uneducated or poor women. The ranks of non-attenders were further swelled during the 1960s by immigrants from the West Indies and the Indian subcontinent, who often found the health-care system unsympathetic to their needs even when they could speak sufficient English to access it in the first place.

Antenatal classes within the voluntary sector (the National Childbirth Trust and the Active Birth Centre founded in 1980) strove to empower women through woman-centred education, although for the NCT, in particular, striking the balance between encouraging women to challenge their carers and attempting to negotiate with professionals at the national level sometimes proved problematic (Kitzinger, 1990). Provision of antenatal classes within the NHS was based largely on a medical model and involved lecturing women about what would happen to them when they came into hospital to have their babies. As late as 1978, the British Medical Association was still publishing leaflets for pregnant women written in strongly paternalistic tones:

> You are going to have to answer a lot of questions and be the subject of a lot of examinations; never worry your head about any of these. They are necessary, they are in the interests of your baby and yourself and none of them will ever hurt you. (quoted in Katona, 1981, p 26)

Today, most childbirth educators recognize the importance of adhering to an adult education model in the provision of antenatal classes, although training in educating for health professionals appears to be patchy and sometimes inadequate.

CLASS ATTENDERS AND NON-ATTENDERS

The history of antenatal education helps explain the current 'middle-class' profile of women (and men) attending antenatal classes and why they are not the people who, it might be suggested, are most in need of childbirth preparation. Research has clearly identified who class attenders are: in both the statutory health-care and voluntary sectors, the women who come to classes are almost invariably white, from social groups I, II and IIIN, and well educated (Nolan, 1995). The situation is the same in Australia (Redman, 1991; Lumley and Brown, 1993; O'Meara, 1993) and the United States (Sturrock and Johnson, 1990; Nichols, 1995). Women under the age of 25 years are less likely to attend classes than older women. While 32% of women giving birth in England and Wales in 1991 were under the age of 25 (Office of Population Censuses and Surveys, 1991), Nolan's survey (1995) showed that only 16% of women attending hospital classes and 8% of those attending NCT classes were in this age group. Overall, fewer than half the women who receive antenatal care in this country also attend antenatal classes (Hancock, 1994).

Effectiveness of Antenatal Classes: the Research Evidence

Many studies have investigated how satisfied those who do attend classes are with the education they receive, and whether antenatal classes influence the course of labour, its outcome, or the psychological well-being of the mother afterwards. Some authors have been able to show a positive effect of antenatal education. Hetherington (1990) reported a significant decrease in the use of analgesia and a significant increase in the number of spontaneous deliveries amongst a non-typical group of class attenders composed mainly of 'inner-city black mothers' when compared with a matched group who did not attend classes. Redman (1991) found that satisfaction with antenatal classes was high and that the women who attended became more knowledgable about birth and parenting. By the end of classes, they were familiar with a range of support organizations to which they could turn after the birth of their babies. It might be suggested, however, that being well-educated women in the first place, they would have been capable of identifying appropriate support groups without any input from classes. Rautauva's Family Competence Study (1991), a national project carried out in Finland, concluded that women who were well informed about childbirth coped better with labour and had healthier babies than those whose knowledge was less thorough. Rautauva suggested that improving health education for women at risk of giving birth to low birthweight babies might be beneficial, but the study did not enquire whether health education alone would be sufficient to overcome the health hazards of poor social circumstances.

Lumley and Brown's study (1993) found no differences between two groups of women, one attending classes and the other not, in terms of birth events, satisfaction with care received and emotional well-being after the birth. Sturrock and Johnson's study (1990) suggested that class attenders were more likely to have a caesarean section or an assisted delivery than those who did not attend classes, to use narcotics for pain relief and to have a long second stage. This study questioned whether training women in coping strategies for labour suppressed their natural ability to make labour effective and tolerable for themselves. Michel Odent is certainly of the opinion that techniques of prepared childbirth are unhelpful because they invite the woman to control her labour from the higher cognitive centres of the brain, centres that should be quiescent if the lower centres that stimulate the release of labour hormones are to work to maximum effect (Odent, personal communication, 1994).

The influential American childbirth educator, Elizabeth Shearer, questions the validity of most of the studies carried out into antenatal education on the basis that they have failed to distinguish between the different educational approaches and childbirth philosophies of various educators. It is her contention that researchers have failed to control for the large number of variables that must inevitably influence the outcome of classes:

> Almost all studies have made the mistake of treating attendance at classes as a single, uniform intervention, but in reality, childbirth classes vary widely by number of hours, instructor training and sponsorship (e.g. hospital-based versus independent) as well as by goals, focus and content. (Shearer, 1996, p 206)

What do Parents want from Antenatal Classes?

While Shearer's comments may be justified, the research evidence none the less poses a considerable challenge to childbirth educators to identify exactly what it is about their classes that women and the people whom they have asked to be their labour supporters find helpful. Whilst it should be the aim of every childbirth educator to reach out and provide a service to women who are not attracted by formal childbirth preparation classes, the legitimate demands of the women who do attend and expect to participate in a useful learning experience should not be overlooked. The opinions of researchers into antenatal education are almost unanimous in suggesting how classes can be made responsive to women's needs:

> *Women . . . often expressed a wide knowledge gap between what they knew about second stage labor . . . and what occurred. They were surprised by the sensations they experienced, the varying intensity or even absence of the bearing-down urge, and the length of the second stage . . . We conclude that childbirth educators should prepare women more realistically.* (McKay et al, 1990, p 197)

> *A major challenge then for childbirth educators is to find ways of preparing women for the realities of the childbirth experience.* (Beaton and Gupton, 1990, p 138)

> *One of the difficulties in antenatal teaching is providing a realistic idea of a previously unexperienced phenomenon – labour and birth.* (Field, 1990, p 220)

> *Mothers whose expectations of labor are unrealistic have been shown to experience more intense pain than mothers who have more realistic expectations.* (Fridh and Gaston-Johansson, 1990, p 103)

> *Classes were considered least useful as a source of parentcraft instruction.* (Gould, 1986, p 59)

> *The women felt that the teaching in these classes did not prepare them adequately for the experience of labour and coping with the new baby afterwards.* (Hillan, 1992, p 276)

> *The level of skills and confidence achieved did not meet the clients' expectations. Under achievement was evident in relation to knowledge about how best to use the health care system; ability to take care of the baby; information on personal health behaviours; information not being timely and having the confidence to bear a healthy child and make decisions for the family's care.* (O'Meara, 1993, p 218)

> *Men and women . . . identified a multiplicity of postnatal topics they felt should have been covered during their classes.* (Nolan, 1996, p 24)

There is a demand for realism in classes, for childbirth educators to abandon the practice of censoring the information with which they provide women and to let the women themselves decide how much and what they want to know about any particular topic. There is also a suggestion that women and their partners are not being well prepared by their antenatal education for the experience of parenting as opposed to the experience of labour and birth.

Realism

Although childbirth educators may have reservations about giving their clients the full story 'warts and all' about labour and life with a new baby, it is clear from the literature that parents do want to know about the complications that may arise during childbirth and exactly what to expect in the early weeks of parenting. The benefits of anticipating potentially difficult life events have long been identified in the psychological literature. Janis (1958) refers to the 'anticipatory work of worrying' and suggests the value of developing coping strategies in advance of a challenging situation. Such preparation helps preserve mental health both in the short and the long term.

The majority of expectant parents are adults. This may seem an unnecessary statement but childbirth educators must remember that their work is with adults who expect, need, and have the right to take responsibility for their own lives and to make their own decisions. To withhold information or to offer a watered-down version of the facts in antenatal classes is to presume to make clients' decisions for them.

PARENTING SKILLS

It is often assumed that people come to antenatal classes solely to learn about labour, and that pregnant women and their partners, especially those who are about to become parents for the first time, cannot project beyond the birth to the weeks and months afterwards. The research quoted above would suggest that this is not true. Men, in particular, are:

> *eager to acquire knowledge and skills that will prepare them for the immediate postnatal period . . . They are concerned about their partners' needs for physical and emotional support, the effect of the baby on the couple's relationship, and their own adjustment to fatherhood.* (Nolan, 1994, p 28)

Preparation for parenthood must encompass not only discussion of the changes in relationships and lifestyle that will occur after the birth of a baby, but also the practical skills that parents need to care for their baby on a day to day basis. It is not longer justifiable to presume that parents will be taught babycare skills on the postnatal ward; staffing levels are often inadequate to allow midwives to spend time with new mothers helping them gain confidence in handling, changing, bathing and soothing their babies. When asked to evaluate the usefulness of their antenatal classes, parents are very clear about where the shortfall lies:

> *I learnt little about coping with and looking after the baby once it had arrived and staff in hospital only have minimum time to show you how to do things.* (mother who attended hospital classes)

> *More information needed about common changes in babies, e.g. cradle cap, milk spots, wind, colic. More about bathing the baby and how often, etc.* (father who attended hospital classes)

> *I would have liked more preparation for early childcare and for lack of quality time with my partner.* (father who attended NCT classes)

> *Please discuss mother's feelings after the birth – your concerns for the baby, how responsible you feel and how worried you can get about the baby's health – NORMAL feelings! (I felt as if I was getting paranoid!)* (mother who attended NCT classes)

PREPARING PEOPLE FOR AN EXPERIENCE THEY HAVE NEVER HAD BEFORE

The majority of clients with whom childbirth educators work are expecting their first baby. Many will never have held a newborn baby, never have seen a woman breastfeeding, and never have been involved in the care of a very young child. Most will never have been present at the birth of a baby. They may have read about birth or seen births on the television, but, unlike their great great grandmothers, these women are unlikely to have helped another woman in labour and been present at the delivery of her child. The essence of antenatal education is, therefore, to prepare people for experiences of which they have little knowledge, even at second-hand. How can this be done? There are many tools that childbirth educators can use to prepare parents effectively for the transition from pregnancy to parenthood (see Box 1.1).

BOX 1.1 PREPARING ADULTS FOR MAJOR LIFE CHANGES

1. Adults, even young adults, have already acquired a lot of life experience that is relevant to the new situation they are facing. It is important for childbirth educators to draw out and value this experience and to help clients build on it in order to meet the new challenges of birth and parenting.

2. The childbirth educator recognizes that adults know what it is like to be placed in unfamiliar situations and how to devise coping strategies to deal with them.

3. By everything she says or does, a childbirth educator can demonstrate that she has confidence in her clients' abilities and that she sees the solutions to the challenges of labour and early parenting as emanating from them and not from her.

4. Everyone expecting a baby has her or his own ideas about labour and motherhood and fatherhood. These expectations are the material with which childbirth educators work in order to help individuals look ahead and plan appropriately.

5. Parents need to learn *practical* skills for coping with labour and parenthood. Childbirth education cannot be just about feelings and physiology. Giving birth and looking after babies are intensely physical activities and childbirth education needs to acknowledge this through the kind of learning activities that it provides.

PHILOSOPHY OF THE BOOK

This book is founded on the author's belief that childbirth education can make a significant difference to people's experience of birth and early parenthood. The research that has been carried out has not pinpointed what that difference is and has not measured it in statistical terms, but the many childbirth educators who are committed to the work they do, who establish short- and long-term relationships with the parents they teach, and who listen to the feedback that parents give them about their classes, are convinced that childbirth education is a force for change. Education is about change – in attitudes, feelings, ability to cope and range of skills. These changes are not imposed on parents by childbirth educators, but come out of the increasing understanding that parents gain through classes of the nature of birth and early parenting. This book espouses the philosophy that education is best understood when it is seen as a process of 'leading forward' (from the Latin: 'e – duco'). What childbirth educators can *tell* parents is probably very little; but the scope for confidence building, for promoting self-esteem, and for helping people devise their own strategies to meet the challenges of birth and parenting is immense.

KEY POINTS

1. Antenatal education aims to help pregnant women (and their partners and supporters) acquire knowledge of childbirth and parenting which,

historically, women acquired from attending births and being closely involved in caring for new babies within their immediate communities.

2. The women (and their companions) who attend classes are generally white, middle class and educated; poor women, women from minority ethnic groups and those less socially privileged and educated rarely attend classes.

3. The literature suggests that what class attenders want is realistic preparation for childbirth and parenting.

4. The life experiences, insights and coping strategies that parents-to-be bring to classes are the tools the childbirth educator uses to help prepare them for the new experiences of labour and parenting.

REFERENCES

Beaton J and Gupton A (1990) Childbirth expectations: a qualitative analysis. *Midwifery* **6**: 133–139.

Dallas (1989) Introduction to: Llewelyn Davies (1915) *Maternity: Letters from Working Women*. London: G. Bell and Sons.

Field PA (1990) Effectiveness and efficacy of antenatal care. *Midwifery* **6**: 215–223.

Fridh G and Gaston-Johansson F (1990) Do primiparas and multiparas have realistic expectations of labor? *Acta Obstetricia et Gynecologica Scandinavica* **69**: 103–109.

Gould D (1986) Locally organised antenatal classes and their effectiveness. *Nursing Times* **82**(45): 59–61.

Graham H (1977) Images of pregnancy in antenatal literature. In Dingwall R, Heath C, Reid M and Stacey M (eds) *Health Care and Health Knowledge*, pp 15–37. London: Croom Helm.

Hancock A (1994) How effective is antenatal education? *Modern Midwife* **4**(5): 13.

Hetherington SE (1990) A Controlled Study of the Effect of Prepared Childbirth Classes on Obstetric Outcomes. *Birth* **17**(2): 86–90.

Hillan E (1992) Issues in the delivery of midwifery care. *Journal of Advanced Nursing* **17**: 274–278.

Janis IL (1958) *Psychoanalytic and Behavioral Studies of Surgical Patients*. New York: John Wiley.

Katona CLE (1981) Approaches to antenatal education. *Social Sciences and Medicine* **15A**: 25–33.

Kitzinger J (1990) Strategies of the early childbirth movement: a case study of the National Childbirth Trust. In Garcia J, Kilpatrick R and Richards M (eds) *The Politics of Maternity Care*, pp 92–115. Oxford: Clarendon Press.

Llewelyn Davies M (1915) *Maternity: Letters from Working Women*. London: G. Bell and Sons.

Lumley J and Brown S (1993) Attenders and Nonattenders at Childbirth Education Classes in Australia: How do They and Their Births Differ? *Birth* **20**(3): 123–130.

McKay S, Barrows T and Roberts J (1990) Women's views of second stage labor as assessed by interviews and videotapes. *Birth* **17**(4): 192–198.

Mead M (1943) *Coming of Age in Samoa: A Study of Adolescence and Sex in Primitive Society*. Harmondsworth: Penguin.

Nichols M (1995) Adjustment to new parenthood: attenders versus non-attenders at prenatal education classes. *Birth* **2**(1): 21–26.

Nolan M (1994) Caring for fathers in antenatal classes. *Modern Midwife* **4**(2): 25–28.

Nolan M (1995) A comparison of attenders at antenatal classes in the voluntary and statutory sectors: education and organizational implications. *Midwifery* **11**: 138–145.

Nolan M (1996) Antenatal education: failing to educate for parenthood. *British Journal of Midwifery* **5**(1): 21–26.

Oakley A (1976) *Housewife*. Harmondsworth: Pelican.

Oakley A (1984) *The Captured Womb*. Harmondsworth: Pelican.

Office of Population and Censuses and Surveys (1991) *Birth Statistics*. London: HMSO.

O'Meara C (1993) An evaluation of consumer perspectives of childbirth and parenting education. *Midwifery* **9**(4): 210–219.

Priya JV (1992) *Birth Traditions and Modern Pregnancy Care*. Shaftesbury: Element.

Rautauva P, Erkkola R and Sillanpaa M (1991) The outcome and experiences of first pregnancy in relation to the mother's childbirth knowledge: The Finnish Family Competence Study. *Journal of Advanced Nursing* **16**: 1226–1232.

Redman S, Oak S, Booth P, Jensen J and Saxton A (1991) Evaluation of an Antenatal Education Programme: Characteristics of Attenders, Changes in Knowledge and Satisfaction of Participants. *Australia and New Zealand Journal of Obstetrics and Gynaecology* **31**(4): 310–316.

Shearer E (1996) Randomized trials needed to settle question of impact of childbirth classes. *Birth* **23**(4): 206–208.

Sturrock WA and Johnson J (1990) The Relationship Between Childbirth Education Classes and Obstetric Outcome. *Birth* **17**(2): 82–85.

FURTHER READING

Chertok L (1969) *Motherhood and Personality*. London: Tavistock Publications.

Dick-Read G (1942) *Childbirth Without Fear*. London: William Heinemann Medical Books.

Lamaze F (1958) *Painless Childbirth: Psychoprophylactic Method*. London: Burke.

2 Antenatal Education: Adult Learners

EDUCATION, NOT INDOCTRINATION

The adults who attend antenatal classes come from complex social networks; they lead lives that touch on the lives of many others and they are engaged in a variety of relationships. Each has experienced many significant life events already and has coped with the inevitable changes and crises that growing to maturity and functioning as an adult entail. Adult learners are, therefore, not blank sheets for the educator to write on; nor do they need others to take control of their lives:

> *The learner is self-directing. In fact, the psychological definition of adult is 'One who has arrived at a self-concept of being responsible for one's own life, of being self-directing.' When we have arrived at that point, we develop a deep psychological need to be perceived by others, and treated by others, as capable of taking responsibility for ourselves.* (Knowles, 1984, p 9)

The knowledge, skills and insights that each adult gains from antenatal education will be set within the context of his or her life, moulding the model he or she has of childbirth and parenting. Whatever the background of the childbirth educator – whether she is herself a mother who has experienced labour, whether she is a midwife or a health visitor or a physiotherapist – the ways in which she has approached or would approach the challenges of labour and parenting are not relevant to the people with whom she works in antenatal classes. It is never appropriate for a childbirth educator to try to impose her own ideas on her clients; this is when education becomes indoctrination:

> *To show someone a new set of rules, tactics and criteria for judging which clarify the situation in which he or she must act is significantly different from trying to engineer learner consent to take the actions favoured by the educator with the new perspective.* (Mezirow, 1983, p 135)

To avoid the trap of indoctrination, the childbirth educator needs to understand her own prejudices about birth and parenting, to acknowledge them, and then to put them to one side so that she can listen without bias to what her clients tell her about their understanding of birth and parenting.

PREJUDICES

Prejudice needs to be thought of by educators in very broad terms: it is, in effect a mind-set or series of mind-sets which are the sum of the cultural indoctrination undergone by the educator

---

BOX 2.1 DISCOVERING YOUR OWN PREJUDICES

Complete the following sentences quickly. You are not trying to give the 'politically correct' answer, but to write down your immediate, uncensored reactions. When you have finished, have a look at what you have written, preferably with a colleague or friend who can help you understand what are the prejudices or stereotypes that, consciously or otherwise, inform your work.

Couples who live together without being married are ....

Pregnancy is ....

Labour is ....

A woman who returns to paid work after her baby is born is ....

A lesbian couple who choose to have a baby are ....

A disabled couple who choose to have a baby are ....

Abortion is ....

A couple who have six children are ....

A couple who choose a home birth are ....

A woman who is frightened of giving birth at home is ....

A woman who wants an epidural for labour is ....

Obstetricians are ....

Midwives are ....

Childbirth educators are ....

Having a baby is ....

Bringing up children is ....

A woman who puts complete trust in health professionals is ....

A man who does not want to be present at his baby's birth is ....

Mothers are ....

Fathers are ....

Parents of a disabled baby are ....

---

as a child, the experiences that she has had during her life and the constraints imposed on her by whichever organization employs her to provide childbirth education. If these prejudices are not to prevent her from offering equal access to learning opportunities for all the clients attending her classes, or to inhibit the clients from making their own decisions about what will be best for them in labour and the early weeks of parenting, the educator must identify, scrutinize and understand her prejudices.

Every childbirth educator needs ongoing opportunities to debrief her own labours, if she has experienced labour, and the labours she has attended. She also needs to debrief her own experiences of being parented, of parenting and of observing other people as parents. Only when she is quite clear in her own mind about the factors that may influence the way in which she handles material during classes is she ready to help adult learners explore on their own terms the new challenges they are facing.

It is possible to listen well (and teaching adults involves at least as much listening as talking) only if the educator is not constantly censoring, either aloud or in her own mind, what she is hearing from her clients ('That's not right!', 'If I were her, I'd . . .', 'Where did he get that idea from . . .?'). The educator helps people to think for themselves when she starts from where they are at in their lives and not from where she is at in her own. (See Box 2.1)

Midwives, physiotherapists and health visitors may approach classes with a feeling that they need to prepare people for the realities of hospital policies rather than simply provide them with unbiased evidence and allow them to form their own opinions about the merits of various ways of managing labour. Educators working within the voluntary sector may believe that they need to stick to the 'party line', which perhaps promotes breastfeeding very strongly against mixed or bottle feeding, for example. Whilst it is quite legitimate to inform parents about hospital protocols and to raise their awareness of the many advantages for mother and baby of breastfeeding, adult education is taking place only when educators present their clients with choices based on the best possible evidence available and leave the decision-making to them. The Baby Friendly Hospital Initiative (World Health Organization/Unicef, 1989) recognizes that adult learners should be able to make an informed choice about infant feeding and does not prevent childbirth educators from discussing bottle-feeding alongside breastfeeding in antenatal classes. Adult learners are, in any case, quick to perceive when they have not been given the full story:

> And when we find ourselves in situations where we feel that others are imposing their wills on us without our participating in making decisions affecting us, we experience a feeling, often subconsciously, of resentment and resistance. (Knowles, 1984, p 9)

ADULTS AS RESPONSIBLE LEARNERS

Adults who seek antenatal education want to prepare themselves for the most important job they will ever undertake, that of bringing up a child. There is no greater influence on the shaping of society than the parenting that its citizens receive. Being a parent means making decisions on behalf of one's children not just many times during their childhood, but many times during each day of their childhood. Antenatal education is essentially about preparing people to make decisions on behalf of vulnerable human beings. It will singularly fail to do this if the educator adopts an authoritarian stance and treats her clients as children who need to be told what they should do rather than helped to understand the relevant issues so that they can choose what will be best for them and their babies:

ANTENATAL EDUCATION: A DYNAMIC APPROACH

If, instead of giving instructions, we give women factual, research-based information about the risks and benefits of all their options, they will be in a better position to make an informed choice and to feel in control, and they will also be more likely to develop confidence and self-esteem. (Schott, 1994, p 3)

Some would argue that there is, in our society, a crisis of dependence on so-called 'expert opinion'. Such dependence is evident when parents turn continually to health professionals for guidance about childbearing and child-rearing. It is not, however, surprising that this should be the case when many new parents receive little support from their own parents or relatives because they live at a long distance from them and when the place of birth has shifted from home to hospital so that most young women have no experience of labour or the first days of parenting:

A young woman today, therefore, has had no early experience with children and has no built-in family supports to assist her in developing her role as mother. The course many women take is to turn to professionals who are presumed to have more under- standing than the young mother of childhood and mothering. (Brazelton and Keefer, 1982, p 96)

Although, in recent years, it has become apparent that expert opinion is often based on little more than custom and practice, prejudice and gut feeling, there is still a need in most people to rely on professionals to make all sorts of judgements and decisions about their lives for them. *A Guide to Effective Care in Pregnancy and Childbirth* (Enkin et al, 1995), which offers a summary of randomized controlled trials in obstetrics, lists amongst 'Forms of care unlikely to be beneficial':

Reliance on expert opinion instead of on good evidence for decisions about care. (Enkin et al, 1995, p 406)

Today, health carers are increasingly aware that 'expert opinion' must take into account the patient's or client's unique understanding of his or her own body and personal circumstances, and that the best health-care decisions are made when a partnership is established between client and carer. Kirkham describes an approach to antenatal education whereby the midwife-teachers abandoned their traditional pedagogic approach and assumed the role of facilitators, inviting mothers and fathers who had just had their babies to lead classes:

We have increasingly encouraged the teaching to be undertaken by the real experts – new parents. (Kirkham, 1991, p 67)

Antenatal education can embody an understanding of how adults learn and reflects the philosophy of contemporary health care when it encourages parents to think for themselves, to discuss issues from their point of view and to devise personal solutions to problems they themselves have identified. Adult learners are each other's best instructors and the role of the childbirth educator is simply to facilitate this reciprocity. By empowering parents to trust their own judgements, antenatal teachers are contributing to the development of a health-care system in which clients can take the responsibility for decisions regarding their own and their children's health:

Antenatal classes have begun to reflect the shift of the focus of care from practitioner convenience to consumer needs, from power-broking to power-sharing, and from directive practice to negotiated practice. With women and their families in the centre, the agenda becomes theirs, and what is valued and meaningful for them is often in sharp contrast to the system's priorities. (Walsh, 1993, p 120)

Learning in Small Groups

Cyril Houle, an influential exponent of adult education, states:

> Adult education is the process by which men and women . . . seek to improve them-selves or their society by increasing their skill, knowledge or sensitiveness. (quoted in Groombridge, 1983, p 3)

Each of the three kinds of learning that he identifies needs to take place in antenatal education: parents must learn how to look after themselves in labour and the practical *skills* of babycare and how to look after their own bodies; they need to acquire *facts*, and they require time to explore their *feelings*. What kind of environment will help such learning take place? Formal lectures given to large numbers of people may increase their knowledge but are unlikely to help them acquire sensitiveness or skills. Increased awareness of one's own and other people's feelings is likely to be acquired only in situations where there can be an exchange of views between people who are comfortable (physically and mentally) talking and listening to each other. Skills are best taught and practised in situations where the instructor can give individual guidance and support to learners. This means, in effect, that adult learning is likely to be most effective when learners come together in small groups with a facilitator.

Box 2.2 Advantages of Small Groups

1. **The childbirth educator can establish an individual relationship with each person in the group, enabling her to become aware of individual learning styles and needs.**

2. **Parents get to know each other when they meet regularly in a small group and can offer each other support during the transition to parenthood.**

3. **Most adults are inhibited by being in a large group. They will offer their opinions on personal or intimate matters only if they know and trust the people to whom they are speaking.**

4. **Small groups enable the childbirth educator to use a variety of teaching approaches: discussion, learning 'games', practical work, role play, brainstorming, buzz groups, case studies, etc.**

This book presupposes that childbirth education is most effective when educator and clients meet in small groups. The group may consist of only two people – the childbirth educator and the mother; or three – the educator, the mother and her partner; or it may consist of nine or ten women or seven or eight couples and the educator. It is not likely that the group will consist of more than 20 individuals, and once it becomes larger than about ten people, the educator will probably find that learning is more effective if she frequently splits the group into smaller groups.

Pregnancy and Learning

Adult educators are often in the privileged position of dealing with people who are highly motivated to learn, who want to participate in their own learning, and who already have considerable skills and insight with which to inform their learning. This is especially true for childbirth educators, whose clients are particularly open to new ideas and willing to reassess their lifestyles:

> Pregnancy is a time of numerous changes in a woman's physical, psychological, and social disposition. These changes, coupled with a desire to have a healthy pregnancy outcome, are powerful motivating forces for women to engage in learning about selected health issues. (Strychar et al, 1990, p 17)

The learning that goes on during pregnancy affects not only the woman who is attending classes, and her partner or chosen companion who attends them with her, but also the next generation as the woman's child becomes the object of the learning she has achieved.

Pregnancy is the time when the woman who is about to become a mother and the man who is about to become a father start to rebuild their image of themselves to incorporate the role of parent. The factors that influence how this happens are multiple. They include the individual's own experience of being on the receiving end of 'good' and 'bad' parenting; role models derived from friends and relatives who are already parents; media images; and encounters with health professionals and childbirth educators. If people are confirmed by health professionals and educators in their new role as parents, they will find it easier to integrate that role into their existing self-concept:

> We can now begin to construct a situation in which a woman can express her own choices and establish her autonomy as a prospective parent. This is not just a simple matter of giving her a feeling of power in the situation. Being autonomous in this uniquely female achievement is paramount to her own development as a woman. The autonomy is necessary to foster the positive side of her feelings of competence as a mother and to allow her to derive self-esteem from the role. (Brazelton and Keefer, 1982, p 101)

The birth of a baby makes particularly real for adults the balance that living in harmony with themselves and other people requires. Perhaps the essence of parenting is creating and sustaining a situation in which parents can fulfil their responsibilities both towards themselves and towards their children. During pregnancy, most people feel a sense of increased responsibility and anxiety about how they will continue to nurture their own individuality alongside caring for their baby. They are open to exploring the boundaries between self and others:

> Since parenthood involves negotiating commitments to self and to others, the dialectic between autonomy and affiliation becomes highlighted around the transition to parenthood. (Fedele et al, 1988, p 96)

This dialectic may be particularly difficult for women because they have traditionally been trained to put the needs of others first. Childbirth education offers the opportunity to women to define the level and type of commitment that is required of them in order to ensure both the healthy upbringing of their child and their own development as separate and uniquely talented individuals. Summarizing the literature that has investigated the psychosocial development of women, Caffarella and Olson (1993) conclude:

> Women's development is characterized by multiple patterns, role discontinuities, and a need to maintain a 'fluid' sense of self. The importance of relationships and a sense of connectedness to others (is) . . . central to the overall developmental process throughout a woman's life-span. Yet, there also appears to be a need for women to capture their own spirit of self, to be given recognition not just for who they are, but for individual abilities and competencies. (p 143)

Aims and Learning Outcomes

Much has been written on the subject of aims and learning outcomes, and devising them has been the task of many educators who have failed to appreciate their significance. It may be quite possible for a childbirth educator to work with groups without having consciously formulated her aims and learning outcomes, but if she is to provide coherent, empowering and effective learning opportunities, she must first have identified very clearly both her aims (what overall it is she hopes to achieve during her classes) and her learning outcomes (what particularly it is she hopes her clients will learn during each class).

Aims

The aims of a childbirth educator embody the *philosophy* that underpins her classes, her one-to-one sessions and every occasion when she works with parents. They describe all the critically important things she hopes to do but which it is virtually impossible for her to know that she has achieved, such as helping parents to understand themselves better; minimizing feelings of guilt where guilt is inappropriate and unhelpful; empowering people to stand up for themselves; helping them to feel that they are not alone in the challenges they face; reinstating the importance of instincts . . . The aims of a childbirth educator are those benchmarks to which she refers every time she facilitates an activity in her classes, initiates a discussion amongst her clients, or demonstrates and encourages parents to acquire practical skills for labour and parenting. Aims are essentially non-specific and couched in abstract terms, and have the zeal of a campaigner about them. (See Box 2.3)

BOX 2.3 AIMS OF CHILDBIRTH EDUCATION

- **To build parents' confidence and self-esteem**

- **To enable parents to make informed choices**

- **To enable parents to communicate effectively with health professionals**

- **To increase awareness amongst women of their own bodies, feelings and needs**

- **To enable women to achieve physical and mental health after childbirth**

- **To increase awareness amongst women's partners and labour supporters of their feelings and needs**

- **To enable women's partners and labour supporters to achieve mental health after childbirth**

- **To encourage parents to take responsibility for their own health and the health of their babies**

- **To encourage critical thinking about medical interventions in order to protect the normality of birth and the right of consumers to receive only evidence-based care**

- **To create a positive sense of group identity so that parents' experiences and feelings can be validated by sharing them with others**

Although childbirth educators are likely to share many aims in common, each will express them in a way that is unique to her. It is likely that one childbirth educator will look at the aims of another and feel in sympathy with them whilst wanting to question a particular emphasis or a certain choice of word or phrase that does not quite reflect her own philosophy of childbirth education. It is therefore important for each educator to draw up her own aims and to revisit them periodically in order to ensure that they continue to reflect her increasing understanding of the needs of adult learners and of parents.

Learning Outcomes

Learning outcomes are far more specific than aims. They are phrased so that the educator can immediately challenge herself as to whether the learning that she hoped would take place did or did not do so. Whereas it is difficult, if not impossible, to test whether aims have been achieved, learning outcomes are, by definition, testable.

When preparing a session, the educator needs to ask herself:

What will my clients have learnt by the end of this session?

Learning outcomes are sometimes described as 'objectives' in the educational literature. Kyriacou (1992) defines them thus:

Educational objectives cannot be stated in terms of what pupils will be doing, *such as working through an exercise, drawing a map or small group discussion. These are activities used to promote learning. The educational objectives must describe what is to constitute the learning. One of the major pitfalls in teaching is to neglect thinking precisely about educational objectives and to see planning as simply organizing activities. While the two go hand-in-hand, it is all too easy to think that a lesson that went well logistically (viz: pupils did what you intended) was effective, until you ask yourself* what the pupils actually learned. (p 23)

Learning outcomes are therefore expressed in far more concrete terms than aims. (See Box 2.4)

There is no escape from learning outcomes. At the end of her session, the childbirth educator asks herself whether they were achieved. If practical work did not take place, or a particular discussion never got off the ground, or vital information wasn't shared or given, the educator must ask herself 'Why?'. (See Box 2.5)

When learning outcomes are not achieved, it is important for the educator to ask herself:

1. What further skills she may need in order to help parents learn effectively.

2. How she can better manage the time she has so that key activities are not missed.

3. Whether she has identified parents' learning needs accurately.

By reflecting on her practice and seeking actively to improve her skills, she will become increasingly able to construct and facilitate sessions in such a way that learning outcomes can be met.

The critical importance of aims and learning outcomes in delivering antenatal education that is responsive to both parents' and facilitators' agendas will be revisited in Chapter 12 when evaluation is discussed. Although the educator may find it challenging and time consuming in the beginning to clarify her aims and learning outcomes, perseverance pays off in terms of enabling her to focus with greater clarity on the provision of effective learning opportunities for parents.

BOX 2.4 LEARNING OUTCOMES

By the end of this session, parents will:

1. Be able to state the pros and cons of gas and air, TENS (transcutaneous electrical nerve stimulation), pethidine, Meptid (meptazinol), epidurals and mobile epidurals.

2. Have developed skills for coping with contractions in late first stage.

3. Understand how a baby moves through the mother's pelvis in second stage.

4. Be familiar with different pushing techniques for second stage and different positions they could use for second stage.

5. Understand the range of feelings they might experience when their babies are born.

6. Have reflected on their own childhood and identified some of the things that contribute to good parenting.

7. Have developed relaxation skills for use in the early days of their babies' lives.

BOX 2.5 WHY WERE LEARNING OUTCOMES NOT ACHIEVED?

SOME SUGGESTIONS

1. *Not enough time.* Was this because people wanted to look at topics that had not been intended for the session (and therefore achieved different learning outcomes from the ones planned)? Or was it because some activities were allowed to go on for longer than was really useful? Or was it because there really was not enough time and fewer topics need to be planned for the next session?

2. *People did not want to do the activities planned.* Was this because they had different priorities from the educator? Or because the activities planned were too difficult or threatening? Or because the educator did not facilitate the activities well?

3. *The educator did not initiate the activities or discussions planned.* Was this because they were too threatening to *the educator*? Or because she changed her session plan in order to meet more urgent needs?

KEY POINTS

1. Adult learners already have considerable knowledge, insight and skills that educators can build on.

2. To enable parents to make decisions that are appropriate for them, childbirth educators must have identified and debriefed their own experiences of birth and parenting, and have confronted their own prejudices.

3. Childbirth educators prepare people for the responsibilities of parenting by building their self-confidence and self-esteem, and helping them to devise coping strategies relevant to their personal circumstances.

4. Adults learn well in situations where they feel free to exchange opinions, share knowledge and practise skills. Small groups provide an ideal learning environment.

5. It is important to understand the role of aims and learning outcomes in constructing teaching sessions that meet the needs of parents effectively.

REFERENCES

Brazelton TB and Keefer CH (1982) The early mother–child relationship: a developmental view of woman as mother In Nadelson CC and Notman MT (eds) *The Woman Patient, Volume 2: Concepts of Femininity and the Life Cycle*, pp 95–110. New York: Plenum Press.

Caffarella RS and Olson SK (1993) Psychosocial development of women: a critical review of the literature. *Adult Education Quarterly* **43**(3):125–151.

Enkin M, Keirse M, Renfrew M and Neilson J (1995) *A Guide to Effective Care in Pregnancy and Childbirth*, 2nd edn. Oxford: Oxford University Press.

Fedele NM, Golding ER, Grossman FK and Pollock WS (1988) Psychological issues in adjustment to first parenthood. In Michaels GY and Goldbery WA (eds) *The Transition to Parenthood: Current Theory and Research*, pp 85–113. Cambridge: Cambridge University Press.

Groombridge B (1983) Adult education and the education of adults. In Tight M (ed.) *Adult Learning and Education*, pp 3–19. London: Croom Helm.

Kirkham M (1991) Antenatal learning. *Nursing Times* **87**(9): 67.

Knowles M (1984) *Andragogy in Action*. London: Jossey-Bass.

Kyriacou C (1992) *Essential Teaching Skills*. Hemel Hempstead: Simon and Schuster Education.

Mezirow J (1983) A critical theory of adult learning and education. In Tight M (ed.) *Adult Learning and Education*, pp 124–138. London: Croom Helm.

Schott J (1994) The importance of encouraging women to think for themselves. *British Journal of Midwifery* **2**(1): 3–4.

Strychar IM, Griffith WS, Conry RF and Sork TJ (1990) How pregnant women learn about selected health issues: learning transaction types. *Adult Education Quarterly* **42**(1): 17–28.

Walsh D (1993) Parenthood education and the politics of childbirth. *British Journal of Midwifery* **1**(3): 119–123.

World Health Organization/Unicef (1989) *Protecting, Promoting and Supporting Breast Feeding: The Special Role of Maternity Services*. Geneva: WHO.

3 Constructing a Course of Classes Part 1: Practical Arrangements and Teaching Approaches

VALUING THE TRADITIONAL ANTENATAL COURSE

The traditional course of antenatal classes is only one of many educational opportunities available to the childbirth educator. It is none the less a very valuable one, offering men and women the chance to build up a substantial knowledge base over a period of time and to work through their feelings, and giving childbirth educators the chance to refine their group-work skills and receive feedback from people who have become familiar with their teaching style.

Whilst the people who attend antenatal courses organized along traditional lines represent a fairly narrow section of society, their power to influence 'the system' should not be under-estimated. They are often the people whose life experiences have given them the confidence to ask for what they want and to question their care. They may well be the kind of people whose self-esteem is sufficiently high to enable them to exercise fully the ideal of 'informed choice'. It is they who give feedback to providers about the quality of the service being provided.

It would be a shame if current efforts to bring antenatal education to the hard-to-reach groups meant that the development of quality antenatal courses for traditional class attenders was overlooked. For the childbirth educator, the insights to be gained from a series of classes in which she can really get to know the parents attending and facilitate an ongoing, in-depth exploration of labour and parenting are considerable. The continuity of carer which an antenatal course run by one childbirth educator provides enables women and their supporters to establish a significant relationship outside the clinical setting.

PRACTICAL ARRANGEMENTS FOR ANTENATAL COURSES

It goes without saying that the practical arrangements that surround antenatal classes have to suit both clients and educators.

Box 3.1 Practical Arrangements – Questions to Ask

1. What kind of lifestyle do the women (and men) who want to attend classes lead? Will they be able to come to classes during the day, or are the majority at work? At what time do they finish work and when would it be reasonable to expect them to arrive at classes?

2. Where is the best place to hold classes, taking into account:

   • safety, especially if classes are held in the evening

   • ease of access by public transport

   • parking facilities

   • ease of access for wheelchair users

   • people's comfort (the size of the teaching room, decor, seating arrangements, floor covering, noise level, lighting)

   • toilet facilities for able-bodied and disabled parents

   • availability of refreshments

   • availability of and storage space for teaching aids

   • cost of hiring the venue?

3. How many sessions should the course include, taking into account that:

   • the longer the course, the greater the commitment required from class attenders

   • there is a lot of material to cover during an antenatal course?

4. How long should each session be, taking into account that:

   • adult learners in general and pregnant women in particular have a limited concentration span

   • people who are attending evening classes, especially if they are pregnant, are soon tired and it is unlikely that much learning will take place after 10 p.m.?

5. Is the course going to be just for women, or for women and their chosen labour supporters? Or will it include some sessions for the women only and some to which supporters can come as well? Will it include a session for fathers to attend without their partners?

6. How many people will there be at each session, bearing in mind that:

   • adults learn best in small groups

   • if people are coming to classes in order to make friends, numbers need to be small enough to make socialising easy?

Inevitably, some give and take will be necessary. The first step towards reaching a mutually acceptable compromise is to ask women and their families what arrangements would best suit them. Questionnaires can be handed out to parents attending antenatal clinics or to those who are already taking classes. The results of such a survey can then be set against what the childbirth educator is reasonably able to offer within the context of her own working and private life.

Often, the times at which classes are run and the places in which they are held are determined more by custom that by finding out what parents would like. An educator in Edinburgh working with a disadvantaged inner city population wondered why attendance at her 5.30 p.m. classes was so poor. When she asked the women, they told her that watching the Australian soap 'Neighbours' was the highlight of their day and there was nothing they would give that up for. The educator moved her classes to 6.30 p.m. and the attendance rate rose immediately. (See Box 3.1)

ADVERTISING

A childbirth educator working with the ex-patriot British community in Belgium wanted to increase attendance at her classes. She discovered that everyone moving to Brussels from the UK received a quarterly mailing from the British Embassy during the first year of their stay. An advert placed in the mailing had an immediate impact on the numbers coming to her classes. Just as the best way to make practical arrangements for classes is by asking parents what they want, so the best way to advertise classes is by using the networks with which parents are familiar. It is important that adverts are well designed and attractive, but even more important that they are seen by the target audience. Finding out which local newspapers women read, which community centres they frequent, and which health clinics and surgeries they attend will identify the best places to put adverts for antenatal classes.

Women and their partners who have signed on for an antenatal course will be under-standably apprehensive about coming to their first class. Some of that anxiety can be alleviated if the educator sends out beforehand a brief welcoming letter, including:

- the suggested content of the course

- appropriate clothing for the women to wear

- whether class members need to bring anything with them such as pillows or mats

- what refreshments will be available

- the facilities on site for disabled people

- clear instructions on how to reach the venue

- a telephone number to contact the educator if the woman or her supporter has a particular concern she or he would like to discuss before the course begins

SETTING THE AGENDA

Committed childbirth educators may consider that there is so much information they would like to share, so many skills they would like to impart and such deep discussions they would like to initiate that even a course of a year's length would scarcely be long enough. However, as antenatal courses are rarely longer than 4–8 weeks, the only way to choose from the multiplicity of topics that could be covered is to ask class attenders to identify those of most importance to them. Learning is most likely to take place when the topics covered in classes are the ones that people want to learn about. (See Box 3.2)

BOX 3.2 SETTING THE AGENDA

Aims

- **to encourage class attenders to take responsibility for their own learning**
- **to boost the self-esteem of class attenders by valuing the topics that are important to them**

Learning outcome

By the end of this activity, class attenders will have

- **identified the topics they want to cover during their antenatal course**

Split the class into small groups of three or four: groups could consist of couples *or* people who have come together could be asked to split up so that each can express his or her views independently *or* class members could be separated into single-sex groups so that both men and women can identify what is important to them.

Ask the groups to discuss what they would like to cover during their antenatal course
or
Ask them to discuss what aspects of labour and caring for their new babies they are particularly worried about.

Let the groups get on with the task; watch discreetly from a distance, ready to intervene when it is apparent that people are running out of ideas and becoming uncomfortable. Watch also for early indicators of who are the more dominant class members and who are the quieter people.

Invite the groups to come together again. Ask for their ideas. Write down *everyone's* contribution on a flip-chart.

If the educator believes that group members are insufficiently at ease to benefit from being split into small groups at the first class, she may choose to brainstorm ideas for the course in the whole group. Although group members will probably put forward their suggestions tentatively at first, provided the educator responds positively to every idea, writing it down on a flip-chart for all to see, other members will feel more confident to contribute.

It is very unlikely that an educator will find class members have a completely different agenda for their antenatal course from what she has anticipated. However, an exercise such as the one described above provides clues as to the relative importance people attach to various topics. One group may be very keen to look at a variety of postnatal issues whereas another would prefer to concentrate mainly on labour. One group may include several members who are likely to need a caesarean section and who want to learn a lot about that and how they will feel afterwards, whereas another might be full of women who have had problem-free pregnancies and whose focus is on how to avoid interventions during labour. If the educator considers that important areas have been omitted from the group's initial agenda, she can either suggest topics herself or ask half-way through the course whether there is anything people want to add to it. Parents and supporters will become more aware of the areas they want to learn about as the course progresses.

Box 3.3 shows an agenda drawn up in 1996 by eight couples attending classes in late pregnancy.

BOX 3.3 WHAT THIS GROUP WANTS TO LEARN

Pregnancy
- How to cope with the discomforts

Birth
- What happens? What is it like?
- How to cope with pain: drugs and self-help techniques
- How to make labour as easy as possible
- Different positions for labour and giving birth
- Breathing techniques
- How to relax
- Water birth
- When to go to hospital

After the birth
- What it's like having your own baby
- How to help a toddler adjust to a new baby
- Baby equipment
- How to look after a baby
- Time management
- How to cope with conflicting advice
- Breastfeeding – how to do it

DEVELOPING THEMES IN ANTENATAL CLASSES

Developing Themes

The joy of running a series of classes for a stable population of group members is the opportunity to develop themes over a period of time. Topics such as 'Stress and Relaxation' and 'Becoming a Parent' can be covered using a variety of teaching approaches from class to class in order to provide people with a structured and empowering learning experience. It is useful for the educator to map out a complex topic in such a way that she can see how best to advance from a basic to a deeper exploration of the subject. Spidergrams are a useful mapping out technique.

Making a Spidergram

Write down the topic in the middle of a blank sheet of paper and circle it. Surround the central circle with smaller circles containing all the ideas that relate to it. Then draw lines between the smaller circles to indicate ideas that seem to be closely linked and should probably be taught together. Finally, number the smaller circles in the order in which they might be covered during classes (Fig. 3.1).

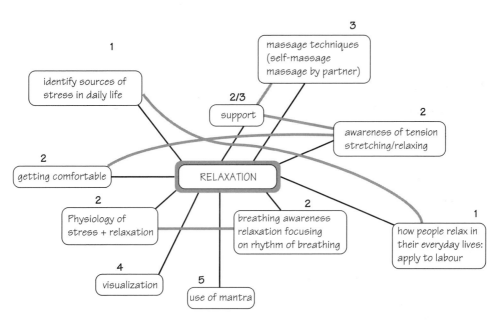

FIG. 3.1   *Spidergram for teaching relaxation in antenatal classes.*

Spidergrams offer a dynamic planning technique because they reveal the multiplicity of links between aspects of a topic. They enable the educator to offer people a comprehensive and integrated learning experience and avoid the trap of putting the course material into 'learning boxes'. (The 'tonight's topic is relaxation' syndrome implies that there will be no need to refer to relaxation again during the rest of the course.)

Balance in Classes

There are all sorts of balances that help to make classes dynamic and effective learning opportunities. The educator is aiming to achieve a balance between:

- parents talking and educator talking
- talking and doing

- people sitting down and people moving around

- labour issues and parenting issues

- topics that are easy to talk about and those that are difficult (e.g. stillbirth and disability)

- whole group work and small group work

- different teaching approaches

Variety in classes helps parents and supporters to concentrate throughout the session, so maximizing the learning they can achieve. Because adults have already developed their own learning styles, the childbirth educator also needs to use a variety of teaching approaches to ensure that everyone has the chance to learn in the way which he or she finds most effective. Educators need to look at the plan for each class and ask:

Are there opportunities in this class for people:

- to learn by listening (either to me or to each other) and by discussing?

- to learn by looking (charts, videos, pictures, etc.) and by handling (model pelvis, baby doll, amnihook, etc.)?

- to learn by doing (either practising skills for labour or for looking after a new baby)?

Is this class:

- going to be lively, varied and stimulating?

If each class contains a balance of listening, discussing, looking and doing, the educator will be sure that each group member has the chance to learn in a way best suited to his or her needs.

Giving and Sharing Information

All pregnant women and all those who come to classes with them have heard, read or seen something about labour, birth and babies. Bearing this in mind, it is far more effective for the educator to use what people already know than simply to offer the same pre-prepared lecture to each antenatal group or each individual parent, regardless of their existing knowledge. Why?

1. People feel valued if the learning they have already achieved is acknowledged.

2. They learn more effectively if new facts are built on and linked to what they already know.

3. Unless people have the chance to share what they have heard, it is impossible to identify whether they have wrong information which needs putting right.

4. Educators can save themselves a lot of time if they avoid giving information that parents already have.

In any antenatal class, it is rarely necessary for childbirth educators to be presenting information for more than a few minutes at a time. Nor is it effective to give lengthy lectures; most people cannot concentrate for longer than 10 minutes and will retain only a very small proportion of what they are told. They are more likely to remember things if they have had the opportunity to learn in a way that enables them to share what they know and to identify and then find out what they want to know.

Sometimes educators find that people know very little about a certain topic: third stage is one example, where universal ignorance seems often to be the norm. In such situations, it is important to think about how the facts can be conveyed in an accessible way:

- Identify beforehand the three things it is most important for parents and their supporters to know about the topic.

- Present information clearly and briefly to group members.

- Ask whether anyone wants further information on the topic.

- Respond to questions.

- Consolidate learning by summarizing the facts, recapping on them at a later class, or devising an activity that involves people making use of the information they have gained.

The information that people retain is the information that is of interest to them. It is therefore more effective to offer basic facts and then to elaborate in response to questions than to offer a great deal of information that may not be perceived by group members as relevant.

Discussions

However experienced an educator becomes, however well she keeps herself up to date, however many people she talks to and listens to, she will never be in a position to understand completely the situation of a single person who comes to her for childbirth preparation. Other than in the rare situation where the childbirth educator herself happens to be pregnant, she is always going to be at a different stage of life from that of her clients. It is wise, therefore, to acknowledge that the best people to identify effective coping strategies for labour, birth and parenthood are the mothers and partners themselves. What the childbirth educator can do is to provide opportunities for parents and their supporters to share their ideas with each other and thereby to clarify and develop them.

Promoting discussion is an essential skill of childbirth educators. There are a number of points to bear in mind:

1. From her very first contact with the group (or with an individual parent or a couple) the educator needs to make it clear that she is interested in hearing their views by asking open-ended questions and listening without interrupting to their responses.

2. People often find it difficult to put forward their ideas in very large groups and may talk more freely if split into smaller groups. Sometimes, however, people in a group that is already fairly small may feel 'safer' talking in the whole group.

3. When working in small groups, class members need to be clear about the work they are being asked to do. It can be helpful for the educator to prepare a sheet for each group with instructions or questions written on it. For example:

- What do you know about breastfeeding?

- What do you think about babies sleeping in the same bed with their parents?

- Which form of pain relief would you prefer to use in labour, or prefer your partner to use?

Some groups find it hard to respond to an open-ended question about feelings, and are more comfortable discussing facts. Discussions that start with people sharing what they know will, however, often develop into discussions about what they feel.

4. The educator needs to listen to whether people are really challenging themselves about the topic they are discussing or are simply skating over its surface. If there is no in-depth exploration going on, she can ask some open-ended questions to encourage people to explore their ideas more deeply.

5. If the discussion is going well, the educator does not need to say anything.

6. Most discussions have a natural lifespan beyond which they become moribund. The educator needs to identify when what is being talked about is merely repetition. This is the cue to bring the discussion to an end.

7. It is important to value what has been discussed by summarizing the main points or asking one of the group members to summarize.

Whilst discussion is generally valuable in any learning situation, it is important to recognize that it is only one way in which people can learn. Some people do not enjoy discussion and consider it a waste of time. Research into education has suggested that there may be differences in the learning styles of men and women:

> *Women have a primary concern with interpersonal relationships which serve as a key source of their self-identity and personal development. Accordingly, women (are) characterised as more able to learn from one another, or in a collaborative mode, than alone or in a competitive mode. Gender (is) assumed to be the basis for this preferred learning style. In contrast, men (are) ... more likely to succeed in competitive or autonomous learning situations.* (Hayes and Smith, 1994, p 212)

Many childbirth educators agree that men enjoy acquiring facts and feel more in control if they have a lot of 'technical' information about a particular topic. Some men (and women) are uncomfortable talking about feelings and may be resistant to learning opportunities that focus exclusively on an emotional agenda. However good a discussion seems to be, therefore, it is important that it should not take the session over to such an extent that other opportunities for learning, such as through practical skills work, are pushed aside.

Learning by Seeing

Many people find that they retain information or an idea more easily if they have not only heard it, but have also been offered a visual image to reinforce it. The most successful visual aids are generally those the childbirth educator has developed or chosen for herself. Visual aids do not have to be expensive but a certain element of creativity about them assists learning. The neck of a polo-neck sweater, for example, can represent the cervix when a doll is placed inside to show how the baby's head helps the cervix to open. A grapefruit can be used to show how easily a baby's head will pass through the pelvis if the mother is in an upright position and not sitting on her coccyx.

There are some key points for the educator to bear in mind when selecting her teaching aids:

- Everyday items are excellent aids to learning.

- Three-dimensional visual aids are always more interesting than charts and posters.

- Visual aids that people can handle and manipulate for themselves are especially useful. A model pelvis passed around the group may help people to understand more about the birth process than many a lecture. Visually impaired parents learn primarily through touch and all their antenatal education should centre on teaching aids that they can handle (Nolan, 1994).

- Charts and posters need to be large, uncluttered and convey only one or two ideas. Few people have the energy to study a densely worded chart or a poster that includes a large number of pictures.

- Writing on a flip-chart creates an on-the-spot visual aid. Group members themselves can be asked to write down key points on the chart (the words they choose are often highly indicative of their understanding of, or attitude towards a particular topic). Or the educator can do the writing, which should be neat and well spaced.

If people are invited to write down the key points that arise during their small group discussions, the childbirth educator can collate them. Handouts based on people's own ideas rather than the educator's are an excellent way of helping them to value themselves and to trust in their own abilities. Handout 3.1 shows a handout which was based on work done in four small groups by class members considering how to meet different people's needs after the birth of a baby.

The best visual aid of all is the childbirth educator's own body. An educator who is suf-ficiently relaxed and confident to point out anatomical landmarks on her own body, to demonstrate good and bad posture in pregnancy and comfort positions for labour, to illus-trate the panting sounds and grunts that women make when having contractions and to show how to position a baby at the breast is continually reinforcing the message that labour and early parenting are physical experiences. So often, childbirth education classes model birth as an entirely cerebral activity; there are plenty of opportunities to talk about what happens, but few to prepare for it physically. Classes that include a large physical skills element, facilitated by an educator who never asks parents to practise anything she has not herself demonstrated first, will inspire confidence in the woman's ability to give birth to her baby.

The childbirth educator can use her own body to:

1. Point out the landmarks of the pelvis – iliac crests, ischial tuberosities, symphysis pubis. Parents will feel free to explore their own pelvis if following the example of the educator.

2. Demonstrate the rocking movements that help the baby's head press down evenly on to the cervix and comfort the woman during a contraction.

3. Demonstrate the different positions that might help a woman labour comfortably.

4. Demonstrate the breathing patterns that might be helpful during contractions, and the panting, pushing and grunting noises that are usual in second stage.

5. Demonstrate how an all-fours position or a hanging squat can help the baby be born gently and minimize the woman's risk of tearing.

6. Demonstrate how to put a baby to the breast 'chest to chest and nose to nipple'.

To be able to use herself as a visual aid, it is important for the educator to feel at ease with her own body. An educator who is not at ease needs to find out why, because it is probably impossible to inspire parents with confidence in the body's ability to give birth unless she is comfortable with her own.

HANDOUT 3.1
Who needs what?

BABY

- Food, sleep, washes, warmth, cuddles, contact, stimulation, clothes

MOTHER

- Reassurance that she is doing a good job (stick with the people who boost your morale and ignore those who don't!)

- Contact with other mothers/adults
    e.g. through Mother and Baby groups, NCT Open Houses, baby clinics, postnatal exercise classes, 'swim with your baby' classes

- Professional help
    GP, Midwife, Health Visitor

- Time for herself

- Time with her partner (without the baby? What about baby-sitters?)

- Food, sleep, practical help

FATHER

- Reassurance that he is a good father

- Not to be pushed aside in favour of the baby

- Contact with supportive adults
    e.g. other fathers, people at work who will listen, friends at home who will listen, health-care professionals

- Time with the baby

- Time for himself

- Time with his partner (without the baby? what about baby-sitters?)

- Food, sleep

© Harcourt Brace and Company Limited 1998

Learning by Doing

If women are to become more confident in their ability to give birth, each antenatal class needs to include a chance to practise physical skills for labour. If the educator is running a series of classes, it is important for her to introduce physical skills work at the first session so that the pattern for future classes is established. The longer it is before people start to practise, the more difficult it will be to overcome their inhibitions and get them out of their chairs. Practising positions for labour or trying out massage or breathing patterns need not exclude women who are disabled if the educator keeps in mind what they are able or willing to do and takes that as her starting point.

Enabling people to practise skills for labour or for looking after their babies depends largely on the confidence of the childbirth educator and her own belief in the value of such practice. If she is not convinced, for example, of the value of offering women the chance to work through a 'practice contraction' by rocking their hips, dropping their shoulders and relaxing whilst their labour supporter massages their shoulders, she is unlikely to facilitate such a learning experience effectively. It is, however, true to say that many childbirth educators who are convinced of the value of practical skills work still find it difficult to handle in classes, and an entire chapter of this book (Chapter 7) considers how to provide effective opportunities for parents to learn physical skills.

Learning with Videos

Most adults today are accustomed to watching videos and may well have been in situations where videos have been used as teaching aids. However, it is possible to run an antenatal class or course without them and videos may simply be a waste of time or even counterproductive if used too much or without careful selection beforehand.

The image on the screen is very powerful. Parents' ideas about what birth is like will be greatly influenced by videos shown to them during pregnancy. The educator should consider what messages any video she might select will send to the particular people who are to watch it. Is the video empowering? Parents need to feel confident and upbeat about labour and birth. On the other hand, if the video shows a woman coping with labour using only her own resources, how will parents feel later if they themselves need to have pethidine or an epidural during their labour? Is the video culturally appropriate? A class that consists entirely of women from an ethnic minority group is likely to dismiss as irrelevant a video showing a birth to a woman from a different ethnic group. Whatever the video the educator selects 'says' about birth, she needs to help parents understand that it portrays only one scenario and that the experience of birth is different for each woman having a baby.

Considerations to bear in mind about videos are:

1. Will the video help parents learn effectively?

2. Is the video to be used

- up to date

- racially, culturally and religiously relevant to the people who will watch it?

3. Will the video make particular parents, for example a disabled woman or a teenage woman, feel excluded?

4. If the video shows a birth, have group members been properly prepared for what they will see?

5. Have people been given the option *not* to see the video if they don't want to?

Videos can certainly help give a realistic idea of birth, but people need to be prepared beforehand for what they will see and debriefed afterwards. If some group members are anxious about seeing a birth on video, but do not want to leave the room, the educator can suggest that they concentrate on one aspect of the video. Focusing on details, rather than the whole, helps to soften the impact. (See Box 3.4)

BOX 3.4 PREPARING TO WATCH A BIRTH VIDEO

The educator may suggest that group members:

• **Look especially at the ways in which the midwife and the woman's supporter help her during her labour.**

• **Note the positions that the woman finds comfortable during labour.**

• **Observe how many people are present in the room when medical intervention is needed.**

There are a number of practical considerations to take into account when planning a session which is to include a video:

• Is there a video recorder and television available for the session?

• Has the room in which the class is held thick curtains to exclude the light?

• Will seating arrangements allow everyone to see the video easily?

• Can the video be set up beforehand so that no time is wasted during the class?

• Will there be sufficient time during the class for the video to be discussed afterwards so that group members are not left with unanswered questions and unexplored fears?

This last point is especially important. Hobbs (1994) describes the power of videos and the need for debriefing afterwards:

> As the pregnant women and their partners watch the tape that you have chosen for them, they can't help but bare open their very souls. Their hearts and minds will be wide open, and to end a video, switch the lights back on and wish them a safe drive home would be the worst thing an educator could do. The teacher needs to delve into that open space within each expectant parent and soothe it. She needs to gently and carefully close it back up before dismissing the group. (p 8)

BEGINNINGS AND ENDINGS

The first class in a series is never easy, either for the group members or for the childbirth educator. People need to be helped to get to know each other so that they can start working together, sharing ideas and exchanging opinions. First impressions are very important:

1. The room needs to be prepared beforehand, with chairs arranged in a circle and tables, if possible, positioned so that class members can put their belongings down.

2. If there are people who are wheelchair users attending, a space in the circle needs to be made ready for them.

3. Each member of the group should be greeted individually on arrival.

4. If the educator starts immediately to introduce people to each other, the more quickly will she and everyone else become familiar with each other's names.

5. Inviting people to make themselves a drink as they arrive gives them something to do – and then something to hold on to.

6. The gap between the first person arriving and the last can be awkward; people can be invited to look at books or leaflets to fill in the time. It is also useful if childbirth educators have a supply of light conversation.

The class needs to start promptly at the time advertised, thus making it clear that punctuality will be a ground rule. As people generally dislike having to come into a room when a session is already in progress, late-comers will hopefully be encouraged to arrive earlier on subsequent occasions. In any case, it is discourteous to keep those who have made the effort to come at the right time waiting for those who are late.

Introductions

If one of the aims of the childbirth educator is to make her classes client-centred and client-directed, it is important for her to hand the class over to the group as soon as possible. The longer she herself talks at the beginning of the first class, the harder it will be for her to get the class members talking.

There are many ice-breaker exercises available; the best ones are those with which the childbirth educator feels most comfortable and which are most effective in encouraging people to talk. (See Boxes 3.5, 3.6, 3.7)

BOX 3.5 ICE-BREAKER 1

Aim

- **to create an atmosphere in which friendships can be made and support networks put in place**

Learning outcome

- **by the end of this exercise, people will know each other's names and where they live in relation to one another**

1. **Using the room to represent the area in which class members live, identify four points in it as towns or villages to the north, south, east and west of the area. Invite group members to stand in the room according to where they live. They will need to talk to each other to position themselves appropriately.**

2. **Ask each person to say where he or she is standing and what their journey to the class has been like.**

BOX 3.6 ICE-BREAKER 2

Aims

- to create an environment in which friendships can be made and support networks put in place

- to encourage group members to take responsibility for their own learning

Learning outcome

- by the end of this session, group members will know each other's names and will have identified for themselves what they want from the course

1. Ask each member of the group to move across the room and talk to the person opposite. Suggest they exchange names, say when their babies are due, how their pregnancies have been, and anything else that occurs to them.

2. Be aware of how people are coping with the exercise and, if one pair seems to be short of conversation, join them to help them out.

3. After about 5 minutes, or earlier if conversation seems to be lagging, invite pairs to join into groups of four.

4. Offer each foursome a piece of paper and ask people to write down what they want from their antenatal course. Set a time limit of a few minutes.

5. Bring all the groups back together and go round the room, asking each person to introduce herself or himself.

6. Ask people to share some of the ideas they have thought about in their small groups regarding what they want from the course. *Wait* for someone to reply. When one suggestion has been made, *wait* for another.

Groups that are very mixed in terms of people's social, racial or religious backgrounds may find ice-breakers that require them to socialize 'instantly' too hard. In such cases, the educator may help group members start to relax with each other by using a non-threatening ice-breaker, perhaps simply asking each member of the group to turn to the person next to him or her and exchange a few words. Finding out what people want from the course can be done in the whole group rather than in small groups (Ice-Breaker 2). If the educator thanks people by name for their contributions, the group members will soon start to get to know each other.

Ice-breakers are not simply for the first session of a course, but for every session. Sometimes, when there is a lot of material to cover during a class, it can be tempting to omit an introductory activity. However, the time spent in helping people get to know each other has a considerable pay-off in terms of one of the principal aims of antenatal classes, that is fostering the development of supportive relationships. The chat that goes on at the start of a class enables group members to relax and prepares them to participate fully in later discussions and activities.

BOX 3.7 ICE-BREAKER 3

Aim

- to create an atmosphere in which friendships can be made and support networks put in place

Learning outcome

- by the end of this session, everyone will have spoken to and know the names of most of the other members of the group

1. Give each person a list as follows:

AUTOGRAPH HUNT

Find someone who: **Signature**

Was born under the same star sign as you

Has visited Italy

Is an auntie/uncle

Reads the same newspaper as you

Watches 'soaps'

Has the same colour eyes as you

Is a vegetarian

Plays a sport

Likes gardening

2. Ask everyone to stand up and complete the exercise by obtaining the signature of one other member of the group against each item.

Introducing Learning Opportunities

When inviting class members to undertake any activity, be it practical skills work, small group discussions or 'games', the childbirth educator needs to ensure that people are quite clear about what it is they are being asked to do or discuss. An activity that seems self-explanatory to the educator because she is very familiar with it may be totally obscure to the group. Therefore, it is important to:

- tell class members why the activity will be helpful to them

- describe what they are being asked to do

- repeat the instructions

- indicate how feedback is to be given (if at all)

- ask whether everyone understands

- move around the room while the activity is being undertaken to answer questions and offer support

When the activity is over, learning can be consolidated if the educator:

- asks people to feed back the main points of their discussion or to describe what they have learned from doing the activity

- asks whether the activity was useful

- summarizes the learning that has taken place

Providing a structure for each learning experience will help parents and their supporters to retain what they have learned and to use their knowledge and skills during labour and birth and the early days of parenting.

Box 3.8 Ending the Course

Aim

- **to boost group members' confidence and morale**

Learning outcomes

Class members will have:

- **consolidated their understanding of the physical and emotional aspects of labour**

    or

- **further developed their relaxation skills**

    or

- **identified their own needs after the birth of their babies**

    or

- **taken one step towards maintaining the antenatal group as a support network**

The educator may:

- **read out an enthusiastic birth report written by a mother or her partner**

- **lead a relaxation which invites class members to visualize holding a sleeping baby**

- **provide an opportunity for parents to exchange ideas about something they enjoy doing now and which it is important for them to make time to go on doing after the birth of their baby**

- **discuss arrangements for people to meet again socially before and/or after the birth of their babies**

Ending Classes and Courses

It is very easy for educators to fall into the trap of leaving 'difficult' topics such as third stage, caesarean section, stillbirth and postnatal depression to the final session of the course. Topics that clients and educators alike find challenging need to be spread throughout the course and preferably introduced at the start of a session so that there is plenty of time for the educator to change the mood and send people away on a positive note.

By the end of the traditional third-trimester antenatal course, labour will be imminent for most of the women in the group and it is important that the final session offers an opportunity for people to recap their knowledge of labour and to practise again the self-help skills they have been learning during previous sessions. (See Box 3.8)

CONCLUSION

Educators who have been leading antenatal classes for many years and those who are just starting work may all have to take a step into the dark in order to provide learner-centred education which respects, values and capitalizes on the learning parents have already achieved during their lives. Those who have been teaching in a different way from what has been suggested in this chapter may be distrustful of new approaches, questioning whether they will really 'work', doubtful of their own abilities to implement them, nervous of failure or of losing control of their classes. Newcomers to childbirth education may have the same emotions because of their inexperience. Both groups of educators have much to offer: the first group has the insights that come with years of contact with parents as learners, the other has a fresh and open-minded enthusiasm. Both groups can be successful as educators provided they are courageous enough to put parents at the centre of their own learning. This is partly a matter of skills, but much more of attitude.

KEY POINTS

1. The practical arrangements for antenatal classes have to suit both clients and educators. The first step towards reaching a mutually acceptable compromise is to ask women and their families what arrangements would suit them best.

2. The only way to select the most appropriate topics from the multiplicity of topics that could be covered during an antenatal course is to ask group members what they most want to learn about.

3. The process of antenatal classes is as crucial as the content; a variety of teaching approaches ensures that learning can be achieved in different ways to suit different learning styles.

4. The best visual aid of all is the childbirth educator's own body.

5. The beginnings and endings of classes play an important part in helping people get to know each other and develop a support network for themselves.

REFERENCES

Hayes ER and Smith L (1994) Women in adult education: an analysis of perspectives in major journals. *Adult Education Quarterly* **44**(4): 201–221.

Hobbs C (1994) Using birth videos to unlock birthing fears. *International Journal of Childbirth Education* **17**(3): 8–9.

Nolan M (1994) Maternity care for the visually impaired. *Modern Midwife* **4**(5): 18–20.

Constructing a Course of Classes Part 2: From Pre-conception to the Postnatal Period

4

Whilst it is essential for the childbirth educator to discuss the agenda for classes with the people who are attending them, she also needs the security of knowing that she has some ideas of her own about appropriate learning opportunities to provide in each session. As she becomes more experienced in running classes for different groups of people, she is likely to become more aware of the topics that are important for parents and their supporters, and increasingly skilled in tailoring teaching approaches to meet learning needs. This growth is bound to happen if the educator is willing and able to reflect on her own practice, to receive feedback from and exchange ideas with parents and other educators, and then to devise strategies for improving her classes (see Chapter 12).

In drawing up a plan for each class, it is helpful for the educator to begin by considering what learning outcomes she hopes people will achieve during the session, and then to proceed by defining the content of the class and thinking about the teaching strategies she can employ to enable each group member to learn in an enjoyable way. Finally, she needs to check that the learning opportunities planned for the session contribute towards the achievement of her global aims as a childbirth educator as she has defined these for herself.

Antenatal classes are traditionally provided in the third trimester for women who are close to childbirth. This is because the pioneers of antenatal education, people such as Dick-Read, Lamaze and Chertok, considered that its purpose was to increase the confidence of women in the ability of their bodies to give birth, and to raise their awareness of how they could help themselves to ease the pain of labour and cooperate with their carers. Today, we need to have a far broader concept of childbirth education so that it is able to embrace the educational needs of children and young people who might in the future choose to become parents, the needs of women and men thinking about having a baby, the needs of couples who have just become pregnant, and the ongoing and urgent needs of parents who have already had their babies. This chapter offers some suggestions to help educators devise lively and relevant learning opportunities for different groups of people. Class outlines are presented with their aims and learning outcomes, proposed content and some ideas for teaching approaches. They are not a blueprint for 'how to do it', but models that the educator can adapt to suit clients' learning needs and preferred learning styles.

PRE-CONCEPTION EDUCATION

Pre-conception education, it might be argued, can never be started too early. For example, there is a place for letting small children watch and talk about breastfeeding as early as possible so that they internalize ideas about what constitutes *normal* infant feeding. Childbirth educators can work with breastfeeding mothers and teachers to provide opportunities for children in primary school to think about what babies need and how they fit into families. Older children in secondary school can benefit from health promotion education which relates lifestyle to healthy childbearing, and from gaining insight into the practical and emotional adjustments that starting a family necessitates.

Model for Pre-Conception Education

Target group: young people in years 10 or 11 at school

Number of sessions: one 2-hour class

Aims

- to increase young people's understanding of the relationship between a healthy lifestyle and healthy childbearing

- to increase young people's respect for and confidence in the birth process

- to enable young people to develop a realistic view of early parenting

Learning Outcomes

By the end of this session, the class members will be able to:

- describe what constitutes a healthy diet and lifestyle before and during pregnancy

- state the risks of alcohol, smoking and drugs to unborn babies

- discuss the significance of folic acid for the healthy development of unborn babies

- describe how being overweight or underweight affects a woman's capacity to conceive a baby and sustain a pregnancy

- state the dangers of rubella and the possible hazards of the workplace for pregnant women

- identify their own fears in relation to labour and birth

- describe the care required by a new baby

Class Content

Topic: Welcome and Introductions (5 minutes)

Childbirth Educator to introduce herself and say a little about her work.

Ice-breaker questions to the group:

1. What do you know about the way in which you yourselves were born?

2. Do you know where you were born?

3. Were you breastfed or bottle-fed?

4. What impressions have television programmes given you about having a baby?

Topic: Lifestyle – Diet, Alcohol, Smoking and Drugs (20 minutes)

Activity:
Invite group members to write down quickly everything they have eaten and drunk since this time yesterday.

Ask:
Would any of the things you have written down be harmful to a woman who was pregnant?
Would you need to add anything to your diet if you were pregnant?
What would be the most difficult thing for you to change about your diet if you were planning to have a baby?
What do you know about drinking and smoking during pregnancy?
Would you be happy to take any tablets or medicines prescribed for you by a doctor while you were pregnant?
How might street drugs affect your baby if you were pregnant?

Topic: Lifestyle – Relaxation (35 minutes)

Activity:
Educator to invite everybody in the group to indicate on a large outline of a person which parts of the body are affected by stress.
   Make the point that every part of the body is affected by stress and that babies, born and unborn, may be affected by their mothers' stress.

Brainstorm:
How do members of the group relax?

Ask:
Do you think parents with a new baby have much time for relaxing?

Activity:
Lay out a chart with 'Baby's Day' written at the top and 'Mother's Day' written at the bottom. In between are sections for each hour of the day. Eight different-coloured piles of cards represent four activities of the baby and four activities of the mother:

   baby: feeding
            awake/playing
            being washed/changed
            sleeping

   mother: household work/shopping
            preparing food/eating
            sleeping
            time for herself, with her partner

BABY'S DAY

Baby Feeding	Baby Awake/Playing	Baby Wash	Baby Sleeping		
Baby sleeping	MIDNIGHT		Mother sleeping		
Baby feeding	1 A.M				
Baby sleeping	2 A.M		Mother sleeping		
Baby sleeping	3 A.M		Mother sleeping		
Baby feeding	4 A.M				
Baby sleeping	5 A.M		Mother sleeping		
Baby sleeping	6 A.M		Mother sleeping		
Baby wash	7 A.M		Mother preparing food/eating		
Baby feeding	8 A.M				
Baby awake/playing	9 A.M				
Baby feeding	10 A.M		Mother household tasks/shopping		
Baby wash	11 A.M				
Baby sleeping	MID-DAY		Mother preparing food/eating		
Baby feeding	1 P.M				
Baby sleeping	2 P.M		Mother sleeping		
Baby feeding	3 P.M				

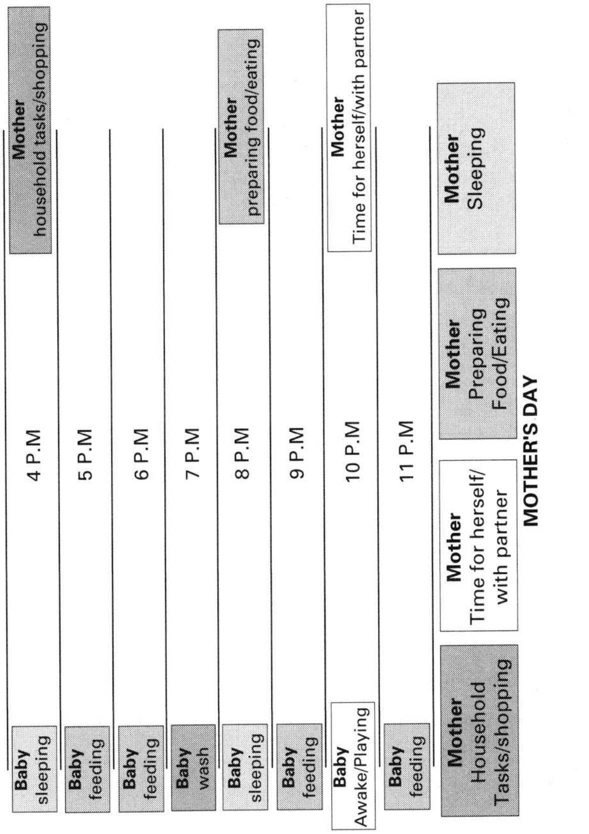

Baby
sleeping — 4 P.M — **Mother** household tasks/shopping

Baby
feeding — 5 P.M

Baby
feeding — 6 P.M

Baby
wash — 7 P.M

Baby
sleeping — 8 P.M — **Mother** preparing food/eating

Baby
feeding — 9 P.M

Baby
Awake/Playing — 10 P.M — **Mother** Time for herself/with partner

Baby
feeding — 11 P.M

MOTHER'S DAY

| **Mother** Household Tasks/shopping | **Mother** Time for herself/ with partner | **Mother** Preparing Food/Eating | **Mother** Sleeping |

FIG. 4.1 *'Baby's Day' and 'Mother's Day' 24-hour chart.*

Invite eight group members to lay the cards out on the 24-hour chart, starting with the activities of the baby.

Ask:
How much time does the mother have for herself? (Or her partner if s/he is the one looking after the baby?)
How might this make her feel?
What would she need to help her cope?

Activity:
Invite the group to participate in a simple, short relaxation exercise, focusing on stretching and relaxing muscles in the face, shoulders and hands.

Break

Topic: Labour, Birth and Pain (10 minutes)

Ask:
What would worry you most about labour and giving birth?

Presuming that the answer is 'pain', ask:
Can someone tell me what the worst pain they have had was?
What did the pain tell you about your body? (that it was injured)
What does labour pain tell you about your body? (that it is functioning normally)

Give information as needed about the pain of labour:

- It tells the mother that her labour has started and she should look for a safe place for her baby to be born.

- It tells the mother how far on in labour she is.

- It tells her when to push her baby into the world.

- It tells her that her body is functioning properly.

Topic: Mechanics of Birth (25 minutes)

Activity:
Invite class members to locate landmarks on their own pelvis (crests, tuberosities, symphysis, coccyx)

Demonstration:
Using a model pelvis and doll, show how the baby moves through the pelvis during labour.

Ask:
What do you think the mother could do to help her baby be born more easily?

Activity:
Invite group members to try out some different positions that might be comfortable for labour.

Ask:
What else might help a woman cope with the pain of labour?

Discuss:

- support from her partner or a friend

- massage

- care provided by health professionals

- a pleasant environment

- relaxation techniques

- medical forms of pain relief

Show pictures of newborn babies and their parents.

Ask:
How do you think a mother and her partner feel when their baby is born?

Topic: Conclusion (5 minutes)

Ask:
Have you any questions you would like to ask?
How do you feel about labour and birth after this session?

EARLY PREGNANCY EDUCATION

Pre-conception education can solve one of the problems generated by the way in which childbirth education is currently provided, namely that third trimester classes are not the time to be offering parents important information about how diet and lifestyle influence the early development of the unborn child. Even early pregnancy courses for women who have just had their pregnancy confirmed are generally too late to be useful in helping them make decisions about how to provide the optimum intrauterine environment for their babies. Early pregnancy courses have, however, an important role to play in helping women and their partners make choices about screening and diagnostic tests and about where they want their baby to be born.

Model for Early Pregnancy Education

Target group: women in the first trimester of pregnancy, preferably before 10 weeks' gestation.

If the women are accompanied by their partners or supporters, the learning opportunities described below can be adapted to include them. For example, men can discuss how they are coping with their partners' pregnancy problems and share their own anxieties about the pregnancy; everyone can usefully learn pelvic floor muscle exercises as part of a healthy lifestyle.

Number of sessions: two 2-hour classes

Aims
- to enable the women to anticipate and therefore plan for the physical and psychological demands of pregnancy

- to promote early mother–infant bonding

- to empower women to make informed choices with regard to pregnancy screening

Learning Outcomes
By the end of these classes, participants will:

- be able to describe how the baby grows and develops during pregnancy

- know some simple comfort measures for coping with pregnancy aches and pains

- have identified for themselves the advantages and disadvantages of home and hospital birth

- know what are the different kinds of care available during pregnancy, labour and the postnatal period (midwife only, shared care, consultant care, etc.)

- have identified for themselves the pros and cons of breastfeeding and bottle-feeding

- understand the difference between a screening test and a diagnostic test

- understand the importance of their pelvic floor muscles and have acquired skills of exercising them

- understand the importance of relaxation and have acquired some simple relaxation skills

Session Outline: Class One

Topic: Welcome (5 minutes)

Childbirth Educator to introduce herself and say a little about her work. Invite each group member to introduce herself and to say a little about how the pregnancy has been so far.

Topic: Pregnancy Discomforts (20 minutes)

Brainstorm:
What sorts of problems do women sometimes have during pregnancy?

List responses on a flipchart. Invite group members to share ways in which they are currently coping with sickness, backache, tiredness, etc.

Topic: Pre-eclampsia (10 minutes)

(This topic leads on from the discussion of pregnancy problems and ensures that women have information about pre-eclampsia at the beginning of their pregnancy.)

Ask:
What do you know about pre-eclampsia?

Consolidate the information group members already have and extend it as required to include the possible symptoms and warning signs.

Topic: Caring for your Back and Pelvic Floor Muscles During Pregnancy and Life (25 minutes)

Show an anatomical chart of a heavily pregnant woman. Ask group members to identify womb/uterus, neck of the womb/cervix, umbilical cord, afterbirth/placenta, bladder, back passage, vagina, spine, etc.

Ask:
What parts of the body come under a lot of strain during pregnancy?

Invite the group to stand and participate in some practical work:

- Show group members how to stand properly in order to protect their backs during pregnancy and for the whole of their lives. (See Chapter 6: Box 6.6)

Using a model pelvis, show where the pelvic floor muscles are located and ask whether group members know why it is so important to keep these muscles strong.

- Invite group members to lean on to the back of a chair with their arms straight. Talk through a pelvic floor muscle exercise routine. (See Chapter 6: Box 6.8)

Ask:
How often do you think you should practise these exercises?
How can you help yourselves remember to practise?

Coffee break (10 minutes)

Topic: Place of Birth (15 minutes)

Invite the women to split into small groups. Ask the members of each group to discuss where they would like their babies to be born and what they see as the advantages and disadvantages of home and hospital birth.

Ask each group to share a couple of its ideas and write them down on a flipchart.

(If this is a couples session, follow the above by inviting partners to spend 3 minutes sharing their feelings with each other about where their baby should be born.)

Topic: Choices about Type of Care during Pregnancy, Labour and the Postnatal Period (10 minutes)

Ask:
Who do you want to care for you during your pregnancy?

Discuss people's preferences and ensure that everybody understands what choices are available locally.

Topic: Relaxation (20 minutes)

Have ready a large outline of the human body. Hand out marker pens and invite group members to indicate on the outline the parts of their bodies that are affected when they become stressed. People might like to draw the sensations they feel.

Using the drawing, point out that stress affects every part of the body.

Ask:
How might a woman's stress affect her baby during pregnancy and labour?

Ask:
How do you relax?

Introduce relaxation exercise by explaining that many people do not recognize that they are in a continual state of stress and that it is important to be aware of how muscles feel when they are tense and how they feel when they are relaxed so that we can monitor our own tension.

Invite everybody to join in a relaxation session. Give people permission not to participate, but ask them not to distract others. Acknowledge that it is difficult to relax in a room full of strangers.

Talk the group through a relaxation session which starts by focusing on the rhythm of breathing and thinking 're' on the in-breath and 'lax' on the out-breath. Then ask group members to:

- pull their shoulders up towards their ears and then relax them

- pull their shoulders down and then relax them

- pull their shoulders back and then relax them

- drop their head forwards on to their chest and then lift it up gently

- drop their head to the right side and then lift it up gently

- drop their head to the left side and then lift it up gently

- frown and then relax all the facial muscles

Ask group members to become aware of how they feel now that the muscles that are often tense are relaxed.

Ask people to focus again on the rhythm of their breathing.

Wait for a few seconds before inviting group members to open their eyes and have a stretch.

When everyone is alert again, ask:

- How did that feel?

Topic: Conclusion: (5 minutes)

Explain that there will be another opportunity to practise relaxation at the next session which will also include discussion of pregnancy screening, clinic visits and baby feeding.

Session Outline: Class Two

Topic: Welcome (10 minutes)

Ask:
How have things been since our last meeting?
Go round the group, inviting a response from each person. Discuss anxieties and problems, and share ideas for coping with discomforts of early pregnancy.

Topic: Antenatal Check-Ups (15 minutes)

Brainstorm:
What examinations do you have during your antenatal visits?
List on flipchart.

Explore with group members the importance of these tests referring back to the discussion about pre-eclampsia in the previous session.

Topic: Antenatal Screening (30 minutes)

Ask group members to name the different kinds of pregnancy tests that are used to assess whether the baby has developed normally.
List them on a flipchart.

If needed, offer brief details about when each test is carried out, how, and what it can tell parents about their baby.

If needed, explain the difference between a screening test and a diagnostic test.

Invite the group to split into smaller groups and ask each small group to discuss one or two of the tests and how they feel about them.

Pool ideas in the large group.

Ensure that the discussion includes what group members would do if a screening/diagnostic test suggested/confirmed that there was a problem with their baby.

Topic: Relaxation Exercise (5 minutes)
(A short exercise such as this can help lighten the mood and enable group members to switch off from one topic in preparation for another.)

Ask group members to stand and:

- take a deep breath in and relax as they breathe out

- roll their shoulders forwards and then backwards

- drop their heads on to their chests and raise them gently

- imagine a string attached to the middle of their scalp pulling them gently upwards so that they are standing tall and straight and feel that their lungs can expand freely.

Coffee break (10 minutes)

Topic: Introduction to Infant Feeding (30 minutes)

Explain that many people make up their minds about how they will feed their babies very early in pregnancy, so now is a good time to discuss feelings and share information about bottle-feeding and breastfeeding.

Ask:
Has anyone definitely made up their minds yet about how they will feed their baby?
Why have you reached the decision you have?

Brainstorm:
Advantages and Disadvantages of Bottle-feeding and Breastfeeding.

Using two sheets of flipchart paper, ask one person from the group to write down pros and cons of bottle-feeding and one to write down pros and cons of breastfeeding.

Ask:
Do you know how you were fed as babies?

Demonstration:
Using simple visual aids such as a balloon and a sock, and group members' own thumbs and forearms (see Chapter 5), help people to understand the difference between feeding from a teat and from a breast.

Information giving:
Explain how breastfeeding works in terms of supply and demand.

Practical work:

- Give several people dolls and ask them to hold the doll as if they were going to bottle-feed a small baby.

- Explain how this position is not appropriate if the baby is going to breastfeed.

- Help group members to position their 'baby' correctly at the breast: chest to chest and nose to nipple.

Discussion:
Are there any situations in which you would find breastfeeding or bottle-feeding difficult?

Topic: Relaxation (10 minutes)

Introduce by linking successful feeding to the mother's (or her partner's) enjoyment of feeding their baby. Babies can sense when parents are tense.

Invite the group to participate in a relaxation session, focusing on relaxing whilst feeding a baby.

POSTNATAL EDUCATION

Perhaps the time when childbirth education is currently most needed is in the early *postnatal* period. *Ante*natal classes are generally ineffective in helping pregnant parents prepare for the early days and weeks of their babies' lives (see Chapter 1). The reason for this may simply be lack of time for childbirth educators to provide learning opportunities about postnatal life as well as covering all the issues that people want to discuss around labour and birth. The way ahead may be to provide postnatal classes for parents to attend with their babies.

The argument against postnatal classes has tended to be that they always start too late to help women and men through the critical early stages of the transition to parenthood. Because this is true, there must always be a place for postnatal topics in antenatal classes. There is, however, an urgent need for ongoing education for parents with young babies, perhaps in the form of a roll-on–roll-off course which women (and members of their families) could start to attend with their babies as soon as they felt ready. Each class would have a designated topic, and parents might choose to attend just one or two classes of the course or every class, and might even repeat the course if it met their need for companionship and stimulation.

Aims, Learning Outcomes and Suggested Content for a Postnatal Course

Target group: parents with babies up to 6 months old. This is a roll-on–roll-off course and parents are welcome to attend any or all of the sessions as soon after the birth of their babies as they feel ready. (Teaching approaches are not included as there are many ideas in this book for covering the topics suggested, see particularly Chapter 8.)

Number of sessions: four 2-hour classes

Aims:
- to increase parents' confidence and ability to make decisions that are right for them and their babies

- to increase the support available to parents during the early months of their babies' lives

- to promote parents' physical and mental health, and thereby, the physical and mental health of their babies

Class One: Learning Outcomes
By the end of this class, group members will:

- have a better understanding of what happened during their labours and of their own emotional reactions during and after them

- have identified their feelings about their choice of infant feeding method and be able to cope with feeding problems

- be familiar with up-to-date thinking about when and how to wean a baby

- have devised strategies, relevant to their personal circumstances, for balancing their needs with their babies' needs

- have acquired some skills of baby massage

Class One: Content

- labour debriefing

- feeding your baby: highs and lows

- weaning: why? when? how?

- sleeping: babies' and parents' needs

- relaxing with your baby: baby massage

Class Two: Learning Outcomes

By the end of this class, group members will:

- understand the range of feelings that parents may experience during the early weeks of their babies' lives and have identified how they themselves are feeling

- know about sexual difficulties that may occur after childbirth and have some ideas about how to overcome them

- be able to state the pros and cons of various contraceptive methods

- know some ways of coping with stress in their daily lives

Class Two: Content

- recovering physically and emotionally after pregnancy and childbirth

- is there sex after birth? joys, problems and possible solutions

- contraception

- parents and their lifestyles – keeping healthy

Class Three: Learning Outcomes

By the end of this class, group members will:

- know how babies develop from birth to 1 year old

- be able to recognize signs of illness in their babies

- have devised strategies for making the home environment a safe one for babies

- be able to state what is the current vaccination programme for babies in the UK

- have identified any problems they are experiencing as parents and have devised strategies for coping

- have acquired skills to help them relax with their babies

Class Three: Content

- how babies develop from birth to 1 year old
- recognizing and responding to baby illness
- safety in and out of the home
- immunizations: when? what? to have or not to have?
- keeping a balance – your needs as a parent/partner/individual
- relaxation session

Class Four: Learning Outcomes

By the end of this class, group members will:

- know what are the nutritional and developmental needs of babies from 6 to 12 months
- have developed skills of stimulating and playing with their babies
- have identified for themselves the pros and cons of going back to work
- know what to ask their employers to provide so that they can continue breastfeeding after returning to work
- be able to describe what options for babycare are available locally, how much they cost and how to access them
- have devised strategies for balancing the demands of work and home
- know what kinds of support are available to working parents

Class Four: Content

- older babies: 6–12 months
- playing with your baby
- feelings about going back to work
- babycare arrangements
- balancing work and home: stress management

'REFRESHER' COURSE

Childbirth educators may be asked to run a 'one-off' session or a short course for a particular group of people such as parents expecting their second or subsequent baby.

Model for a 'Refresher' Course

Target group: parents who have given birth before and are now expecting another baby

Number of sessions: two 2-hour classes

Aims

- to enable parents to use their previous experiences of giving birth and early parenting to help them make informed choices around the birth of their next child

Learning Outcomes

By the end of these classes, group members will:

- have a deeper understanding of their previous experiences of labour, giving birth and early parenting

- know what they would like for their next labour

- have consolidated their knowledge of the birth process

- have acquired self-help skills for labour and birth

- have ideas about how to help their children accept the new baby

Session Outline: Class One

Topic: Welcome and Introductions (10 minutes)

Childbirth Educator to introduce herself and then invite each person in the group to spend a couple of minutes chatting to someone he or she does not already know.
Invite everyone to say his or her name and something about how the pregnancy has been so far.

Topic: Setting the Agenda (10 minutes)

Brainstorm:
What areas do you want to cover during this course?

Topic: Labour Debriefing (30 minutes)

In single-sex groups, invite people to spend 10 minutes discussing what was good about their previous labours and what they would have liked to be different.

Pool ideas in the large group.

Ask partners to work together for 5 minutes, each telling the other how they feel about their previous experiences of labour and birth.

Topic: Summary (10 minutes)

Ask:
Can you summarize the ways in which your previous experiences of labour and birth could have been made better?

List everyone's ideas on the flipchart.

Coffee Break (10 minutes)

Topic: Overview of Labour (25 minutes)

Drawing on people's experiences, briefly outline what happens during first, second and third stage. Discuss with the group what self-help skills were useful at each point.

Using the pelvis and doll, help group members to consolidate their understanding of the benefits of upright positions for labour.

Practise positions for first stage and for giving birth.

Topic: Relaxation (25 minutes)

Ask:
Were you able to relax during your previous labours?
Was being relaxed helpful?
Do you practise relaxation techniques as part of your everyday lives?

Draw out group members' ideas and summarize them in the context of the physiological and psychological benefits of relaxation.

Invite group members to participate in a relaxation session. Focus on helping people become aware of their own bodies and of how each part of their body feels; suggest that people use the rhythm of their own breathing to help them relax, dropping their shoulders and letting go of their tension each time they breathe out.

Session Outline: Class Two

Topic: Welcome (10 minutes)

   Ask group members to say their names and to mention one thing that has stuck in their minds from the previous session.

Topic: Communicating with Staff and Informed Choice in Labour (35 minutes)

Brainstorm:
Ask group members to suggest ways in which they can play an active part in their own care during labour.

Invite group members to split into smaller groups and to list all the questions they would want to ask about any intervention they were offered during labour.

Bring the small groups back together and pool everyone's ideas. (See Box 4.1)

BOX 4.1 INFORMED-CHOICE QUESTIONS
(TO ASK WHEN DECIDING ABOUT INTERVENTIONS IN LABOUR)

- Is this an emergency or do we have time to talk?
- What are the benefits of this procedure?
- What are the risks?
- If we go ahead with it, what other procedures might we need as a result?
- What else could we try?
- What would happen if we waited an hour or two?
- What would happen if we didn't have it at all?

Ask the whole group:
What makes it difficult for you to ask for what you want in labour?

Topic: Relaxation in Labour (15 minutes)

Invite group members to participate in some quick relaxation techniques which could be used between contractions (see Chapter 7).

Ask couples to work together while they imagine having a contraction. Ask the women to tell their partners ways in which they can help.
(Ensure that the women's supporters are caring for their own backs if they are massaging their partners or supporting them physically.)

Talk the group through two or three contractions with brief relaxation periods in between.

Coffee Break (10 minutes)

Topic: A New Family Member (30 minutes)

Invite group members to split into small groups and discuss what they are looking forward to about having a new baby in the family and what they are anxious about.

After 10 minutes, ask each group to share one thing they are looking forward to and one thing they are anxious about.

Invite each small group to look at strategies for coping with one of the things they are worried about.

Pool ideas.

Topic: Relaxed Parenting (20 minutes)
Drawing on the work the group has just done, discuss the benefits of relaxation in the context of parenting young children.

Ask:
What has been your worst moment with the child/ren you already have?

Invite ideas for coping with the stresses of caring for new babies and small children.

Invite everyone to participate in a relaxation session.
During the session, invite group members to visualize coping with a crying baby, a demanding toddler and a messy house. Suggest that they ignore the mess, cuddle their baby, and sit the toddler next to them on the couch with a toy or a book. Suggest that, as everyone relaxes, the tension in the household is diffused.

Offer people the opportunity for a private word if they still have questions they would like to ask.

Eight-Week Third-Trimester Antenatal Course

Planning a long course is as challenging as planning a short one; it is just as important to keep a balance between information sharing and giving, discussion and practical skills work in order to sustain group members' enthusiasm for the course and to provide a range of learning opportunities to suit everybody's style of learning. There follows a brief outline of an 8-week antenatal course. Many ideas for teaching the topics suggested can be found in this book.

Aims, Learning Outcomes and Suggested Content

Target group: women in the late second or third trimester of pregnancy and their partners or supporters.

Number of sessions: eight 2-hour classes

Aims

- to build parents' confidence in their ability to give birth and parent their children

- to enable parents to make informed choices around labour, birth and early parenting

- to increase parents' awareness of their own bodies, feelings and needs so that they can achieve positive physical and mental health during and after the birth of their babies

- to create a positive sense of group identity so that parents' experiences and feelings can be validated by sharing them

Class One: Learning Outcomes

By the end of this class, group members will:

- be familiar with the names of other people in the group

- have identified what they want to learn during the course

- understand how pregnancy has affected them as individuals and as a couple

- know how the mother's uterus and pelvis and the baby work together to help the baby to be born

- understand the importance of relaxation in everyday life and in labour

- have acquired some basic relaxation skills

Class One: Content

- welcome and introductions

- housekeeping (location of toilets, refreshments, facilities for disabled group members, etc.)

- setting the group's agenda for the course

- physical and emotional effects of pregnancy

- how the pelvis works and a brief overview of labour

- introduction to relaxation for labour and life

Class Two: Learning Outcomes

By the end of this class, group members will:

- know each other's names

- have some ideas of how to cope with the discomforts of late pregnancy

- be able to exercise their pelvic floor muscles and stand, get up from bed, and lift things safely

- be able to state the early signs of labour

- have identified how they would like to manage their labour

- be able to communicate their needs to professional carers

- have consolidated and extended their relaxation skills

Class Two: Content

- welcome and round robin: 'tell us what you already know about your baby'

- late pregnancy problems: caring for your back and pelvic floor

- onset of labour

- when to go to hospital (or call the midwife) and what to take (or have available at home)

- knowing who the health professionals are and communicating with them

- birthplans and choices in childbirth

- relaxation session

Class Three: Learning Outcomes

By the end of this class, group members will:

- be able to communicate with their partners in order to ensure that, after their baby is born, everyday tasks are allocated in a way both feel happy with

- know what questions the midwife will ask them and what examinations she will carry out when she arrives at the house or meets them in hospital

- know what are the different kinds of monitoring and the pros and cons of each

- understand the range of hopes and fears that are typical to people facing labour

- have acquired self-help skills for the first stage of labour

- have developed relaxation skills appropriate for labour

Class Three: Content

- welcome and introductory activity focusing on partners sharing the workload postnatally: 'who will be doing what after your baby is born?'

- admission procedures

- monitoring: at home and in hospital

- fears and hopes about labour and birth

- first stage of labour: what happens and how you might feel

- self-help strategies: positions, massage, breathing awareness, relaxation during and in between contractions

Class Four: Learning Outcomes

By the end of this class, group members will:

- know what kind of care is required by premature babies and what facilities are available in Special Care Units

- have consolidated their knowledge of what happens in first stage and have further developed appropriate self-help skills

- know what interventions might be suggested in first stage and how to obtain information from their carers in order to be able to give informed consent

- understand the changes in their relationships and lifestyle that might occur after their babies are born

- be able to list a range of support groups they could access as parents

Class Four: Content

- welcome

- premature babies

- review of first stage

- more practice of self-help skills for first stage

- interventions in first stage: induction, acceleration, artificial rupture of membranes

- changes in lifestyle after the birth of a baby

- 24-hour clock: life with a baby

- postnatal support: professional and lay

- relaxation session

Class Five: Learning Outcomes

By the end of this session, group members will:

- know what are the medical forms of pain relief available in labour and the pros and cons of each

- have identified their feelings about drugs in labour

- be able to describe how labour progresses from transition to the birth of the baby

- have acquired self-help skills for second stage and understand their rationale

- understand the range of feelings experienced by parents when their babies are born

- know what newborn babies look like

- have acquired skills of holding, soothing and interacting with a newborn baby

Class Five: Content

- welcome

- medical forms of pain relief: gas and air, transcutaneous electrical nerve stimulation (TENS), pethidine, epidurals

- transition

- self-help for transition

- second stage: what happens and how you might feel

- self-help skills for second stage

- feelings when your baby is born

- appearance of your newborn baby

- holding and soothing your newborn baby

Class Six: Learning Outcomes

By the end of this class, group members will:

- have a deeper understanding of their own feelings about infant feeding
- understand the principle of supply and demand in relation to breastfeeding
- be able to position a baby at the breast correctly
- understand the reasons and know some possible solutions for common breastfeeding problems such as engorgement and sore nipples
- have identified social attitudes towards breastfeeding out of the home
- be able to relax whilst breastfeeding

Class Six: Content

- welcome
- advantages and disadvantages of breastfeeding and bottle-feeding
- breastfeeding: how it works – supply and demand
- positioning your baby at the breast
- troubleshooting: dealing with common problems
- social aspects of breastfeeding: any time? anywhere?
- relaxation session visualizing feeding your baby

(This class touches only briefly on bottle-feeding as many childbirth educators and health professionals consider that to teach bottle-feeding in antenatal classes is contrary to the spirit of the International Code of the Marketing of Breast-Milk Substitutes (World Health Organization, 1981) and to the Baby Friendly Hospital Initiative [WHO/UNICEF, 1989].)

Class Seven: Learning Outcomes

By the end of this class, group members will:

- have consolidated their knowledge of second stage
- have developed further their skills for labouring in second stage and giving birth
- be able to state the pros and cons of forceps and ventouse from both mother's and baby's points of view
- know the reasons for, procedures during and postnatal care after a caesarean section
- be familiar with the range of feelings experienced by parents whose babies have been born by assisted delivery
- know what happens during a managed and a physiological third stage
- be able to change a baby's nappy, bathe and dress a baby
- know how to protect their babies from cot death

Class Seven: Content

- welcome
- recap on second stage
- assisted deliveries: forceps, ventouse, caesarean
- feelings of disappointment or failure in relation to labour and birth
- third stage
- changing nappies, bathing and dressing your baby, and putting your baby down to sleep

Class Eight: Learning Outcomes

By the end of this class, group members will:

- know the normal physiological changes that occur after birth
- understand the difference between 'baby blues' and postnatal depression
- have identified some of the possible causes of postnatal depression and know the range of treatments available
- have identified the pros and cons of being a working parent
- have further developed self-help skills for labour
- know that they have the option of maintaining the antenatal group as a support group after the birth of their babies

Class Eight: Content

- welcome
- recovering after the birth
- postnatal depression – in men and women
- going back to work: advantages, disadvantages, coping strategies
- 'labour rehearsal': review of what happens and practical skills for coping with contractions
- birth story
- date for reunion

KEY POINTS

1. Having a plan for each teaching session enables childbirth educators to feel confident that they can provide a well structured learning experience whilst incorporating group members' own agenda.

2. Planning teaching sessions means considering the learning outcomes that parents want to achieve, defining the content of each session, and devising teaching strategies to enable group members to learn in an enjoyable and effective way.

3. **Childbirth education today is a broad field covering education in schools for parenthood, education during early and late pregnancy, and the ongoing education of parents who have already had their babies.**

REFERENCES

World Health Organization (1981) *International Code of Marketing of Breast Milk Substitutes.* Geneva: WHO.

WHO/UNICEF (1939) Protecting, promoting and supporting breast feeding: the special role of maternity services. Geneva: WHO.

5 Making the Baby 'Real' in Antenatal Classes

GETTING 'REAL' ABOUT BABIES AND PARENTING

The 'reality' of babies for many women and couples who are pregnant for the first time is composed of images derived from the media and their own fantasies. Whereas 70 years ago almost every young woman would have had experience of holding and caring for a young baby, the women who are today's typical antenatal class attenders may well have had very little such experience or none at all. Although intellectually, parents-to-be are aware that babies are demanding and cry and need feeding day and night, they are dazzled and misled by the plump, clean and smiling babies who regularly appear on our television screens to help boost sales of everything from toilet rolls to cosmetics. Whilst no-one would wish to deny parents-to-be their joyful anticipation of their new baby, an essential part of antenatal education must be to help prepare them for the reality of life after birth.

As long as parents conceptualize their baby in terms of an advertising ideal, there can be no real bonding. There is a grave danger that the contrast between parents' image of their 'perfect baby' during pregnancy and the reality of the baby who is placed in their arms after a possibly long and painful labour will be so stark as to cause considerable emotional upheaval. The transition to parenthood is most easily achieved when pregnant parents are helped to identify with their baby as a unique individual and to anticipate in some detail the kind of lifestyle that goes with new babies.

Making the baby 'real' in antenatal classes starts with the way in which childbirth educators talk and encourage parents to think about labour. It is easy for antenatal classes to isolate labour from its endpoint – the birth of a baby. Thinking about the pain that might be experienced during labour, learning about the ways in which labour can be managed medically, making decisions about who should be present during labour – all these issues can crowd out of the minds of class attenders the centrally important issue, which is that labour culminates in the birth of a baby and that the birth of a baby heralds a new phase in the life of his or her parents.

At the heart of antenatal education lies the challenge of focusing parents on the baby for whom they will soon assume 24 hours a day responsibility. No aspect of pregnancy, labour or the postnatal period should be discussed without reference to the baby. Each time a childbirth educator has contact with a pregnant woman and her partner, she is aiming to strengthen the relationship between them and their baby, and to enhance their confidence to care for him or her after the birth.

The importance of the influence that antenatal education can have on the experience of early parenting should never be underestimated. Setting antenatal education in the broad context of *preparation for parenthood* as opposed to the narrower one of *preparation for birth* helps educators appreciate the impact that their work may have on the way in which society functions.

TALKING ABOUT 'YOUR BABY'

Babies in antenatal classes are variously described as 'the bump', 'bump', 'the baby', 'your baby', 'baby', 'it', 'he', 'she', 'he or she'. If educators' aims include:

- promoting bonding between parents and their babies

and

- increasing parents' confidence to care for their new babies emotionally and physically

and

- enabling parents to make their own decisions about how they want their baby to be born and how they want to parent their baby,

it is essential for them to stress that each woman is carrying a baby who is uniquely hers and her partner's; that each woman will give birth to a baby who from the first moments of independent life can distinguish her from other women by her smell and by the sound of her voice; that each mother can soon distinguish the sound of her baby crying from the cries of other babies. In emphasizing the unique qualities of this relationship, it is therefore surely inappropriate for educators to talk about 'the baby' or 'baby' or 'it'. All babies are 'your baby' in that each parent-to-be must apply the knowledge and insights they gain from classes to their particular relationship with their own baby. Every time a childbirth educator refers to 'your baby', she is stressing that the information being shared or the ideas being discussed or the skills being practised are relevant only within the context of each parent's unique experience of her or his own child.

It can be difficult to avoid referring to the baby as 'it'. Educators may use 'he' on one occasion and 'she' on another in order to deal with the gender issue. Giving thought to the matter is essential. Some parents receiving antenatal education will already have found out the sex of their baby and a relaxation session, for example, which refers to the baby as 'she' when they know they are having a boy will jar no matter how sensitively the educator delivers the relaxation session and how pertinent her images are.

DOLLS AS TEACHING AIDS

A doll is probably the most frequently used teaching aid in antenatal education. It can create a powerful image in parents' mind and needs to be chosen and handled appropriately. A doll used to represent the baby in utero needs to be flexible in order to illustrate fetal positions; it has to pass reasonably easily – although preferably not *too* easily – through a model pelvis. Dolls that need a lot of manhandling in order for them to 'be born' do not boost parents' confidence. A doll that is being used to focus attention on postnatal issues needs to be life-size and, if at all possible, heavy enough to approximate a reasonable newborn weight. Dolls with heavy, floppy heads are excellent for helping pregnant parents gain confidence in holding a baby. It is also important to choose a doll of the right colour to be relevant to the women and men attending classes. In groups that comprise people from different ethnic groups, it is appropriate for the educator to have several dolls of different colours.

Some childbirth educators choose always to treat their teaching doll as a 'real' baby; they carry their doll in a Moses basket, tuck it up after using it in classes, and handle it gently and lovingly. Others treat their doll simply as a teaching aid and make no attempt to suggest that parents should equate it with their own real babies. It probably doesn't matter which option is chosen as long as the educator is consistent: a doll treated as a baby must always be treated as a baby; a doll treated as a teaching aid must always be treated as a teaching aid. Loving the doll one minute and abandoning it on the floor the next is disturbing to parents who are building up an image of their own babies.

MAKING THE BABY REAL: TEACHING APPROACHES

Whether a childbirth educator's contact with parents is through classes or during a one-to-one session at an antenatal clinic or on a home visit or in any other setting, what she teaches should always centre on the relationship between mother and baby or parents and baby.

In classes, ice-breakers can be used to help focus parents immediately on their babies.

BOX 5.1 ICE-BREAKER 1

Aim

- **to assist the transition to parenthood by increasing parents' awareness of their relationship with their babies during pregnancy**

Invite each parent to describe one thing he or she has done for their baby during the last week.

Answers might include
- **decorating the baby's room**
- **cutting down on cigarettes**
- **attending an antenatal clinic**
- **talking to the parent of a new baby**

It is now considered that the idea of the baby as 'the passenger' during labour, playing no active part in his or her own birth is erroneous. The baby would appear to have at least some control over the initiation of labour (Bennett and Brown, 1993), and 25 years ago Leboyer described in poetic terms the efforts of the baby to be born:

We have discovered today that the stimulus that sets labour in motion comes from the child, just as the Ancients said it did. And now we know that the child actually does struggle to be born. (Leboyer, 1974; 9th impression, 1983, p 63)

Nor are newborn babies entirely helpless; it has been shown that a newborn baby, if left entirely alone, will crawl to the mother's nipple and latch on to her breast (Righard and Alade,

---

Box 5.2 Ice-breaker 2

Aim

- **to boost parents' confidence that they already know more than anyone else about their babies**

Invite each parent or couple to introduce their baby to the group, describing whether their baby has a nickname, when he or she is wakeful and when quiet, whether he or she gets hiccoughs, likes listening to music, etc.

Box 5.3 Ice-breaker 3

Aim

- **to empower parents by demonstrating to them their instinctive understanding of how to care for their babies**

Pass the doll round the group and invite the parents to show how they would try to soothe their baby if he or she were crying.

The educator can help class members consider holding the doll over their shoulder, sitting the doll facing them on their knee, cradling the doll in their arms, lying the doll face down on their knees, holding the doll face down along one forearm and patting its bottom with their free hand, etc.

1990). Labour may seem much less frightening to the woman if she can think of it as a process in which mother and baby work together (with the encouragement and assistance of supporters and carers) to make the birth as easy and gentle as possible. Explaining to parents that the positions the mother finds most comfortable during labour are likely to be those that make labour least stressful for her baby encourages women to respond to their instincts. Suggesting that women focus on their baby during contractions may increase their awareness of how to work with the baby to make labour as easy as possible. Women who are reminded that it is the most natural thing in the world to rock new babies or small children in order to comfort them are likely to remember to rock their hips during labour, increasing their own comfort and enabling the cervix to dilate evenly.

The language in which the childbirth educator describes labour can reflect the concept of the baby as an active participant in his or her own birth:

- 'Your baby presses down on the cervix in order to open it up'

- 'During second stage, your baby is moving deep into the pelvis'

- 'Your baby wants to be born gently'

- 'Your baby turns her head in order to help her shoulders come through the pelvis'

Childbirth educators can paint a picture of contractions which emphasizes the baby's role in labour:

> Imagine you are having a contraction. Each time you breathe out, drop your shoulders and blow your breath down towards your baby. Imagine your baby's head pressing on to your cervix. Remember that your baby is in labour as well as you. Blow your breath out down towards your baby. This contraction is nearly over. Are your shoulders loose and relaxed so that you are breathing in plenty of oxygen for you and your baby? The contraction's finished now. Relax and let your baby relax.

All interventions during labour can be discussed in the light of their implications for the baby, and from the baby's point of view. It is important that consideration of second stage should embrace not only discussion of what happens and of how the mother can work with her body to maximize her pushing efforts, but also the moment of birth itself. The emphasis that the

---

BOX 5.4 ROLE PLAY: BIRTH

Aim

- to increase parents' awareness of the complex and divergent emotions that may accompany birth

Learning Outcome

- group members will be familiar with the range of emotions experienced by parents when their baby is born

Invite a woman and her partner or labour supporter to position themselves as they think they might be at the moment of birth. Give the woman a doll to hold as if it were her newborn baby.

Ask the group:

- how the mother might feel? (ecstatic, terrified, exhausted, overwhelmed . . .)

- how her partner might feel? (relieved, protective, tearful, proud, happy, appalled . . .)

- what their baby might be feeling? (relief, terror, calm, excitement, anticipation . . .)

Discuss:

- what the mother might want at this moment? (to be left alone, a cup of tea, to sleep, to gaze at her baby . . .)

- what her partner might want? (to be left alone with the mother and baby, to cry, to rest, to have something to eat, to go and tell everyone about the baby, to go home . . .)

- what their baby might want? (to rest, to stay close to his/her mother, to suckle, to be held and comforted . . .)

---

educator places on the first moments of the baby's life, and the way in which she facilitates exploration of mother's, father's and baby's emotions, helps parents to keep labour in perspective as simply a means to an end. (See Box 5.4)

Parents can also be encouraged to explore birth during relaxation sessions which focus on their babies' feelings. (See Box 5.5)

BOX 5.5 BIRTH: THE BABY'S VIEWPOINT

Aim

- **to increase parents' sensitivity to the needs of their new babies**

Read extracts from poems or books that describe the moment of birth. For example:

Now is the moment.
The baby emerges . . . first the head and then the arms; we help to free them by sliding a finger under each armpit. Supporting the baby this way, we lift the little body up . . . and we settle the child immediately on his mother's stomach . . .
Soon the baby appears to be one breathing mass; one sees the powerful waves course up and down the back, from the top of the skull to the coccyx.
And then, cautiously emerging from under the stomach, an arm, usually the right arm.
The arm stretches out. The hand slides briefly over the mother's stomach, then withdraws.
The other hand ventures out . . . slowly, as if astonished to encounter no resistance, surprised that the space around it is so vast.
And now the legs begin to move. First one, then the other is cautiously extended. Then both begin to kick and thrash, alarmed because they no longer encounter any resistance.
To calm their panic, we can offer them support, the touch of a hand . . .
And then, suddenly, everything moves together, harmoniously. There is no part of the little body that is not involved in this movement.
The baby stretches more and more boldly, thrusting, probing . . .
It's vital to reassure, to pacify the child immediately.
Through her hands, unmoving but tender the mother is saying to her baby: 'Don't be afraid. I'm here. We're both safe, you and I, we're both alive.'

(Extracts from Leboyer, 1983)

It is important to give parents realistic images of what newborn babies look like. Pictures of a baby being born and of babies just a few seconds old are useful, as are pictures that illustrate normal newborn oddities such as milia, swollen genitals, cyanotic hands and feet, and lanugo.

Teaching Babycare Skills

Until recently, a new mother could expect that during her stay on the postnatal ward she would be taught how to change her baby's nappy and how to bathe her baby; if she had given birth at home, the community midwife would have taught her these skills. Today, many women are discharged from hospital within a day or two of giving birth, and overstretched community staff may not see it as part of their brief to help the mother with babycare. Some women may receive assistance from their own mothers, but many look to their antenatal education to equip them with the skills they will need in the early postnatal period.

It is quite clear from the literature that antenatal education often fails to prepare people for the day-to-day management of the physical needs of a tiny baby. When pregnant women are asked what they want from antenatal classes, they will commonly reply along these lines:

General advice on how to care for a new baby in the early days at home.

Anything relevant to bringing up a baby – health care/clothing i.e. amount of clothing/ bathing/temperature for bedrooms etc.

Coping after the birth – feeding/winding/typical medical problems etc. (Nolan, 1997)

There are a number of ways of providing opportunities for parents to acquire babycare skills. The least satisfactory is for the childbirth educator herself to demonstrate, with the assistance of a real baby or a doll, how to change a baby's nappy or how to bathe a baby. Nobody has ever learnt to ride a bicycle by watching someone else; observing a person who is highly competent engage in a practical activity may give some insight into the skills involved, but is no substitute for the learner having a go him or herself.

A new mother and/or father can be invited to visit an antenatal class with their baby and perhaps feed, change and bathe the baby in front of the group. The confidence of pregnant parents is likely to be boosted if they see someone who was, until very recently, as inexperienced as they are, competently undertaking the care of their baby. It is probably unfair to both the visiting mother or father and their baby to ask whether a member of the class can practise changing the baby's nappy and giving a bath. The baby will sense that the person handling her is a stranger and may become unsettled (thus greatly undermining the confidence of the pregnant parent). The pregnant mother or father may be particularly awkward out of a sense of the responsibility of handling someone else's child. One alternative is for class members to practise babycare skills using dolls.

For practise they must: it is impossible to learn how to make Yorkshire puddings by listening to someone describing the process. Only by mixing the ingredients yourself and cooking them do you get a clear idea of what is required. A doll is not a substitute for a baby, but at least it is a three-dimensional object of some awkwardness which can be dressed and undressed by as many parents as needs be.

It is surprising how many questions are generated by practical skills work with dolls. These are questions that group members would almost certainly not have thought of without the stimulus of trying to put a nappy on the doll or hold it with one hand so as to be able to bathe it with the other. There are additional advantages to this kind of class work:

1. If the childbirth educator has several dolls, several parents can 'practise' changing nappies and giving a bath.

2. Even if there are only a couple of dolls per group, the dolls can be passed round so that everyone has the opportunity, for example, to practise holding a baby safely in the bath.

3. Dolls are surprisingly difficult to dress and undress – as are new babies.

4. Men can volunteer (and frequently do) to change and bathe a doll, and they may have even fewer opportunities than women to learn these skills from health carers or grandparents after the birth.

Such a session can cover an immense amount of material in a short period of time. Parents can be helped to think about what equipment is really necessary for a new baby and how many of the things they see in the shops are not necessary at all and perhaps even harmful, such as

---

BOX 5.6 PRACTISING BABYCARE SKILLS

Aim

- to increase parents' confidence in their ability to look after their new babies

Learning Outcome

- group members will be able to bathe a baby safely

Equipment needed:

Several dolls, selection of baby clothes, towels, cottonwool balls, nappy cream, baby soap, baby shampoo, ear buds, selection of nappies, nappy disposal sacks, talcum powder, changing mats, baby baths or washing up bowls

Invite some parents to volunteer to 'bathe' the 'babies'

Ask the rest of the group to guide them through the process

Elicit from the group the following information:

- where to bathe the baby (a warm room)
- choice of baby bath
- how to bathe the baby without straining your back
- items needed (e.g. towels, cottonwool balls, change of clothes, etc.), **not needed** (e.g. talcum powder, ear buds) and controversial (e.g. nappy cream, soap, baby shampoo)
- pros and cons of various types of nappy
- how to bathe the baby, ensuring that she keeps warm (hair and face first while body still wrapped up; then body)
- how to hold a baby safely whilst bathing her
- how long to keep the baby in the bath
- how to dress the baby appropriately for the time of year and the heating conditions in the house
- safe sleeping arrangements for the baby after her bath (following cot death advice)

---

talcum powder. Opinions about the use of baby soaps can be exchanged in the light of individuals' personal or family experience of eczema. Discussion of cot death often arises naturally out of a session of this kind and educators can check that parents are familiar with the most up-to-date guidelines.

Parents enjoy being shown how to play with their babies and learning about 'the amazing newborn' – how a baby tracks, copies facial expressions, and chooses to look at human faces rather than other images. A baby massage demonstration with a real baby gives parents confidence to enjoy their babies and alerts them to possibilities of interaction other than that required simply to meet their infant's basic needs. Whilst these kinds of activity are often overlooked in antenatal classes, they are possibly more valuable in helping parents connect with their babies and laying the foundations for sensitive and enjoyable parenting than any amount of discussion or information giving.

TEACHING ABOUT INFANT FEEDING

Breastfeeding

Just as a childbirth educator needs to have debriefed her experiences of labour, whether her own or assisting at other people's, so she needs to understand her feelings about infant feeding. To avoid sending subliminal messages to parents either pro- or anti-breastfeeding or pro- or anti-bottle-feeding, every childbirth educator should be able to identify her own biases and guard against them. It is important, therefore, for her to find someone who will listen to her while she reflects on how she fed her own babies, if she is herself a mother, and on her observations of other women's infant-feeding practices.

Helping women and their partners and families to learn about breastfeeding is surely one of the most important and satisfying aspects of a childbirth educator's work. Increasing the amount of breastfeeding in our country is probably the single most significant step we can take to improve our health and that of future generations. Sadly, many women have little or no confidence in their body's ability to feed their baby and are victims of prejudices, misconceptions and a great deal of ignorance about how breastfeeding works. Antenatal education aims to help women acquire the knowledge and understanding they need in order to make it possible for them to choose to breastfeed if they so wish. Very often, the hard facts about breastfeeding which remain after the myths have been exploded are sufficiently powerful to encourage women at least to start breastfeeding their babies even if, later, they change to bottle-feeding.

There follows an outline of a 2-hour antenatal session on breastfeeding with a group of women and their male or female supporters. It is not suggested that this outline would be ideal for all groups, but it provides a structure that could be modified to suit the needs of different people and to fit in with whatever time is available to the educator.

Breastfeeding Class

Topic: Introduction – Exploring Feelings About Breastfeeding (10 minutes)

Ask the class:
When did you first see someone breastfeed?
How did you feel about it?

Topic: Advantages of Breastfeeding and Common Concerns (20 minutes)

In small groups, invite class members to:
Write down a list of the advantages of breastfeeding.

BOX 5.7 BREASTFEEDING CLASS

Aims

- to boost parents' confidence in women's ability to breastfeed their babies
- to promote realistic expectations of breastfeeding

Learning outcomes

By the end of this session, group members will:

- know the health benefits of breastfeeding
- understand the principle of supply and demand in breastfeeding
- be able to cite the differences between colostrum and mature milk and between foremilk and hindmilk
- be able to position a baby correctly at the breast
- be able to describe the difference between the way in which a baby feeds from a bottle and from the breast
- be able to describe the baby's likely feeding pattern during the first few days of life and in the longer term
- have identified some of the problems commonly encountered by breastfeeding women and know some strategies for avoiding or coping with them
- know where they can get help if they experience problems with breastfeeding

Visual Aids

- *really good* pictures of babies correctly latched on to the breast
- pictures showing differences in colour and consistency of colostrum, foremilk and hindmilk
- *simple* diagrams to explain the physiology of breastfeeding
- mixture of water and oil coloured with blue food colouring in a bowl and a piece of sponge (see below)
- lots of dolls and pillows
- breastfeeding 'goody bag' (see below)

Articulate any worries they have about breastfeeding.

Pool the ideas that class members have shared in their small groups.

Topic: How Breastfeeding Works (35 minutes)
Explain simply and briefly the physiology of breastfeeding, using charts and pictures to help group members learn.

Give a demonstration of how the composition of breast milk changes as the baby feeds from the breast:

Have ready in a wide-topped bowl a mixture of oil and water stained with blue food colouring. Place three wine glasses on a tray. Dip a piece of ordinary sponge into the oil and water mixture and wait until the sponge is completely saturated. Hold the sponge over the first glass and draw group members' attention to the way in which the water runs out without having to squeeze the sponge. Then start to fill the second glass by exerting a slight pressure on the sponge. Allow a mixture of water and oil to fill the glass until there is more fluid in the glass than in the first. Finally, fill the third glass by squeezing the sponge hard to make the remaining oil come out. The third glass should be less full than the second.

Ask the group to say how they think this demonstration represents breastfeeding. The points to draw out are that:

1. the foremilk is the equivalent of a drink for the baby; it is thin and requires very little effort on the part of the baby to milk it from the breast

2. what follows is a mixture of foremilk and fatty hindmilk; the baby needs to work a little harder to get this from the breast

3. the final part of the feed is the fat-rich hindmilk; the baby needs to suck vigorously to obtain this from the breast

4. some babies may be thirsty again after the hindmilk and may request the second breast after the first is empty in order to have some more foremilk.

Look at positioning a baby at the breast:

Ask people to turn their heads over one shoulder and imagine drinking a cup of tea in that position. Ask them to put their chins down on their chests and imagine trying to drink like that. Then demonstrate with a doll how to hold the baby so that his chest is turned towards the mother's chest and his nose is opposite the mother's nipple and he can feed easily from the breast without having to turn his head.

Invite group members to suck their thumbs, then to suck their forearms (it is impossible to suck a forearm in the same way that you suck a thumb). Explain that this is the difference between the way in which a baby feeds from a bottle and from the breast. Explain the movement of the baby's jaw and tongue whilst breastfeeding.

Give a mother a doll and show her how to hold her baby with her right arm along her baby's spine and supporting his neck if he is going to feed from the left breast and with her left arm along her baby's spine and supporting his neck if he is going to feed from the right breast. Help her to understand that, if she pushes the back of her baby's head on to the breast, his chin will go down on his chest and he will be unable to feed. Explain that she needs to allow her baby to bring his head to the breast himself. The right position is when her baby's spine and the back of his head are in a straight line.

Hand round pictures of babies well latched on to the breast.

Ask fathers and supporters how they think the mother could be made comfortable whilst breastfeeding. Look at choosing a suitable chair to help the mother sit upright and pillows to bring the baby up to the level of her breast.

Invite fathers and supporters to help make the mothers comfortable so that the mothers can practise positioning a doll at the breast. Move round the group answering questions.

Coffee Break (10 minutes)

Topic: Frequency of feeds (10 minutes)
Ask parents and supporters to write down on a piece of paper the times at which they had snacks or meals during the last 24 hours. Ask how many times people had something to eat and how long people had between their snacks. Emphasize the huge variation in the number of times people ate and the length of time between their snacks. Make the point that babies are exactly the same in that some will require lots and lots of small feeds; some will have longer feeds and go for longer in between. Explain that the baby's stomach is about the size of a walnut – it will need filling regularly.

Topic: Strategies for Coping with Problems (25 minutes)
Have ready a 'breastfeeding goody bag' with a collection of items to stimulate discussion about breastfeeding (e.g. hand-held breastpump, breast pads, contraceptives, picture of a screaming baby, nipple cream, nappy, pacifier, cinema tickets, clock, bottle of sterilizing fluid, baggy T-shirt, etc.).

Ask each member of the group to take out an item and say what it makes them think of in relation to breastfeeding. Topics likely to come up are leaking, expressing and storing breastmilk, breastfeeding as a method of contraception, coping with sore nipples, having time for yourself, feeding away from the home, timing of feeds.

Topic: Conclusion – Support Networks (10 minutes)
Ask parents who are the people who will support them when they are breastfeeding.

If the childbirth educator has never herself breastfed, she needs to be particularly aware of the importance of correct positioning of the baby at the breast and to be confident of her ability to teach women a suitable breastfeeding technique. All educators can benefit from:

- asking a Breastfeeding Counsellor or Infant Feeding/Lactation Sister to show her how to position a baby at the breast

- talking to and watching a mother who is successfully breastfeeding her first baby

- practising how to demonstrate breastfeeding while watching herself in a mirror (to get the class members' view)

If the time the childbirth educator has available to teach about breastfeeding is limited, it is important for her to prioritize so that women acquire sufficient knowledge and skill to give them a good chance of breastfeeding successfully. Most people would agree that women need to understand:

1. how to position the baby at the breast

2. that breastfeeding should be baby-led (i.e. demand feeding)

3. that it is important to empty the first breast first

Bottle-feeding

There are many childbirth educators who would favour never mentioning bottle-feeding during antenatal classes. However, because there are serious hazards associated with incorrect bottle-feeding and because many women will, in fact, choose to bottle-feed their babies at some point earlier or later in their babies' lives, it can be argued that to discuss selecting appropriate formula milks and making up feeds is very necessary. Inviting a parent who wants to bottle-feed, or who may choose to use bottles at some point in his or her baby's life, to practise sterilizing a bottle, measuring out formula and adding the correct amount of boiled water will, as with the baby bathing exercise, generate many highly pertinent questions which can be answered by the rest of the group from their own experience, or by the educator.

If it is the policy of the institution or the organization for which the childbirth educator works not to teach parents how to bottle-feed, the educator can help her clients understand how bottle-feeding works by differentiating it from breastfeeding. Thus, at the beginning of her session, she may ask a member of the group to hold the teaching doll in the position he or she would hold a baby if the baby was going to be given a bottle. She can then point out how different this position is from the position the baby needs to be held in if he is to feed successfully from the breast. When looking at the constituents of breastmilk, the educator can remind parents that formula milk is a mixture of chemicals and should be treated as such (i.e. taking great care to measure it out correctly and add the appropriate amount of water). When describing how a breastfeed consists of a drink (the foremilk) followed by a highly nutritious meal (the hindmilk), the educator can point out that breastfed babies do not get thirsty because they have a drink with every meal. She can then help parents understand that a formula feed is 'all meal' and that bottle-fed babies therefore require a drink of cooled, boiled water at least once a day. Parents will then be able to appreciate that bottle-fed babies may get constipated because of lack of fluids but breastfed babies do not get constipated even though they may pass only one or two stools per week. The educator can suggest that the parents of a bottle-fed baby who is crying will need to decide whether he is hungry or thirsty in order to meet his needs appropriately, whereas parents who are breastfeeding can simply offer the breast.

There is also scope for discussing with antenatal groups the pressures of the postnatal ward when bottle-feeding mothers often seem to be finding it easier to placate their babies than breastfeeding mothers. If parents understand the difference between breastfeeding and bottle-feeding, they can project forwards to a few weeks later when the bottle-fed babies may be having problems with constipation, colic or gastroenteritis but the breastfeeding babies and their mothers will have learned how to breastfeed and be finding life much easier. Rather than avoiding the topic of bottle-feeding altogether, which is likely to make parents feel that they are being pressurized into breastfeeding, the educator can make a strong case for breast-feeding by talking about it alongside bottle-feeding. Some parents who were undecided about how to feed their babies may then decide to try breastfeeding because they have been helped to understand that bottle-feeding is not only a less healthy choice for their babies but may not be as easy for them as they had thought.

INVITING NEW PARENTS TO VISIT THE CLASS

It has long been accepted in the literature that patients learn more about the culture and environment of hospitals from other patients than from any health professional who is caring for them (Cormack, 1976). This is true of perhaps all situations in life: those best able to help others through a new experience are the people who have just been through the experience themselves:

> Since the strongest prediction of competence at infant feeding and care was previous experience with infants, both for primiparas and multiparas, the nurse's (childbirth educator's) task of promoting adaptation of the postpartum woman to her role as

mother may be to facilitate opportunities for pregnant women to have contact with other women and their infants. (Salamm, 1995, p 34; author's parenthesis)

We have increasingly encouraged the teaching to be undertaken by the real experts – new parents. (Kirkham, 1991, p 67)

Inviting a woman or a couple who have recently given birth to talk about how they have coped with the first days and weeks of parenting can 'make the baby real' for expectant parents in a particularly powerful way.

The childbirth educator may consider inviting couples to visit whose babies are at different stages of development: a 2-week-old baby looks and behaves very differently from a six-month-old baby, and the parents of each will, in all likelihood, have different feelings about their own competence as parents. It is very encouraging for those who are still pregnant to see how the chaos and strangeness of the early weeks of a new baby's life gradually give way to a routine devised by the baby and his parents which is manageable and familiar to all.

It is vital for the childbirth educator to spend some time beforehand talking to the parents she is inviting to visit the antenatal class. Parents who have had no previous opportunity to talk about their labour and about their life with their new baby may use the class to debrief experiences and feelings that are raw in their intensity. In such a case, the members of the antenatal group will find themselves in the role of counsellors to the new parents rather than in a position where they can learn from the lived experiences of peers who have been able to reflect on and gain insight into the transition to parenthood.

There are a number of points to take into consideration when selecting parents to visit an antenatal class. The childbirth educator needs to ask herself:

- Will these particular parents be comfortable answering questions put by the antenatal group?

- Will they cope with being the centre of attention?

- Have they had the chance to talk about their labours and their early experiences of parenting?

- Will the mothers be happy to feed their babies in front of the group?

- What image of parenting will these parents present?

Some of these questions may sound as if they are designed to ensure that only a sanitized version of reality is offered to the vulnerable pregnant parents in the antenatal group. It is, however, reasonable for the childbirth educator to choose visitors who will offer a balanced account of the first few weeks with a new baby, one in which the problems of colicky evenings and sleepless nights are set alongside the joys of getting to know their new baby and cuddling and playing with him or her. The antenatal group certainly needs to gain an insight into the exhaustion of parenting, but equally into the pride and sense of achievement that it can bring.

In preparing the new parents for their visit, the childbirth educator can discuss:

- whether they are happy to talk about their labours and what they are going to say

- their experiences of early parenting

- whether there are any areas they do not want to discuss (if there are, the antenatal group may need to be steered away from asking inappropriate questions)

- how long their visit is to last (the learning opportunity provided by a visit from new parents is likely to be maximized if the antenatal group knows that it must focus on getting information within a given timespan)

- how their visit is going to be structured (perhaps the fathers speaking to the men and the mothers to the women)

- who is allowed to handle the baby

Often, in a mixed antenatal group, the women dominate and the men, who may in any case believe that theirs is a peripheral role in labour and the early postnatal period, are marginalized and prevented from asking the questions that are important to them. An excellent learning opportunity can be provided by dividing the antenatal class into single-sex groups and inviting the visiting father to talk to the men and the visiting mother to talk to the women. If their consent has been obtained beforehand, the new mother can then talk to the men in the antenatal group and the new father to the women. This enables the women to gain insight into the experience of fatherhood and the men into the experience of motherhood.

The educator can help to generate discussion by writing on a flipchart some questions that class members might like to put to the visiting parents:

- Tell us what your 24-hour day is like.

- For what were you least prepared?

- Did you have help after your baby was born? Who? Was it effective?

- How has your baby changed the relationship between the two of you?

- Did breastfeeding begin as you thought it would?

- What tips do you have for expectant parents?

- What preparations prior to the birth were most beneficial?

(from Tumblin, 1996)

Whatever the new parents say to the antenatal group, their relationship with their baby will become apparent from the way in which they handle her and respond to her. They may be prepared to let their baby be passed round, giving some of the antenatal group their first opportunity to hold a tiny baby. Even if the baby cries continuously or distracts the group from listening to what the new parents have to say, these are learning opportunities in themselves. New babies do cry, and they do attract the attention of other adults (and children). Women often comment on how, whilst they were pregnant, they were the focus of all their friends' and relatives' attention but, since the birth, they have had to take second place to their babies.

After the invited parents leave, the childbirth educator needs to offer the antenatal group a chance to discuss the visit. Whilst a lot of questions will have been answered, it is also likely that some people are dumbfounded by the insight they have gained into the realities of parenting. The childbirth educator can suggest that women and their supporters take a few moments to talk to each other about their feelings and then invite the group as a whole to comment on anything that surprised, worried or encouraged them.

Conclusion

The influence on the antenatal group of a successfully organized visit from new parents can be profound. What the childbirth educator is effectively trying to do is to recreate the social network that once enabled people about to become parents to share in and learn from the experience of people who had recently become parents. No matter how skilled the childbirth educator is as a facilitator, or how recent her own experience of birth and early parenting, what she has to say about babies will never have the same immediacy as the stories of parents who are perceived by the antenatal group to be merely ordinary people like themselves.

KEY POINTS

1. The childbirth educator aims to strengthen the relationship between parents and their unborn babies, and to enhance their confidence to care for their babies after birth.

2. Parents need realistic ideas about what newborn babies look like and how they behave.

3. Teaching practical babycare skills may be more valuable in helping parents connect with their babies and in laying the foundations for sensitive and enjoyable parenting than any amount of discussion or information giving.

4. Childbirth educators need to understand their own feelings about infant feeding if they are to avoid bias.

5. Inviting a woman or a couple who have recently given birth to visit the antenatal class with their baby can 'make the baby real' for expectant parents in a particularly powerful way.

REFERENCES

Bennett VR and Brown LK (1993) *Myles Textbook for Midwives*, 12th edn. London: Churchill Livingstone.

Cormack D (1976) *Psychiatric Nursing Observed*. London: Royal College of Nursing.

Kirkham M (1991) Antenatal learning. *Nursing Times* **87**(9): 67.

Leboyer F (1983) *Birth Without Violence*, 9th impression. London: Fontana.

Nolan M (1997) Antenatal education: failing to educate for parenthood. *British Journal of Midwifery* **5**(1): 21–26.

Righard L and Alade MO (1990) Effect of delivery room routines on success of first breastfeed. *Lancet* **336**: 1105–1107.

Salamm CM (1995) Mothers' perceptions of infant care and self-care competence after early postpartum discharge. *Birth* **10**(2): 30–39.

Tumblin A (1996) A visit with a postpartum couple. *International Journal of Childbirth Education* **11**(4): 16–17.

6 Teaching and Learning About Pregnancy

Classes for parents who have only just become pregnant offer tremendous opportunities for health promotion and should be far more widely available than they are at present. A suggested outline for an early pregnancy class is included in Chapter 4. However, the majority of parents do not start classes until they are in the third trimester of their pregnancies. By this stage, it is too late to cover health promotion topics such as diet, drugs, alcohol and smoking in pregnancy. The time of fetal organogenesis is past and, although parents might benefit from learning about healthy living, their agenda tends to be focused exclusively on how to cope with labour and look after their babies once they are born.

EXPLORING FEELINGS ABOUT PREGNANCY

It is not too late, however, even when parents are heavily pregnant, to help them explore their reactions to the pregnancy, their relationship with their unborn child, and the changes in their perceptions of themselves and their relationships with others. The aims of the childbirth educator when she is facilitating learning about pregnancy in antenatal classes might be summed up as follows:

1. to help parents adapt to their new role as mother/father

2. to enhance the mother's and father's prenatal attachment to their baby

3. to promote positive parenting

The 9 months of pregnancy represent a period in women's and men's lives when their outlook on the world changes to incorporate a stronger sense of responsibility; ideas of personal freedom are revised and priorities reassessed; relationships with their own parents are restructured on a basis of equality rather than dependence.

These changes may not be evident either to themselves or others, or they may manifest themselves very dramatically. One father who recently attended the author's own classes told how he had always been a 'yes man' at work, keen not to rock the boat, prepared to do extra hours if it kept the boss happy. Since his partner had become pregnant, he had discovered within himself a previously unsuspected capacity for assertiveness and was now conducting his working life on an entirely new basis. His wife, on the other hand, very much a woman of the world who had been accustomed to taking the dominant role in their relationship, now described herself as 'completely laid back' and focused, to the exclusion of all else, on her pregnancy.

As parents become more aware of the subtle emotional changes that they are going through during pregnancy, they start to appreciate how profoundly their unborn baby is already affecting their lives. The emotional work of pregnancy is important for a healthy transition to parenthood.

Pregnancy seems to be the most salient time for a full-blown possible parental self to emerge. (Antonucci and Mikus, 1988, p 70)

Antenatal education can help make more conscious and comprehensible the changes that parents are perhaps only dimly aware of going through. The importance of providing education in small 'safe' groups is critical in this context because parents will not share feelings of ambiguity or hostility about their pregnancies in a group which they fear may be judgemental or fail to validate their experiences. The childbirth educator may invite people to share feelings about pregnancy at the beginning of the course and offer further opportunities to talk in later classes when the group is more cohesive and people feel freer to reveal what they may initially have thought were unacceptable viewpoints. (See Box 6.1).

BOX 6.1 HOW DID YOU FEEL WHEN YOU FIRST FOUND OUT YOU WERE PREGNANT?

Aim

- **to raise parents' awareness of their own and other people's attitudes towards pregnancy**

Learning outcome

- **group members will be familiar with the range of reactions to the confirmation of pregnancy**

In small groups or in the whole group, invite class members to discuss how they felt when they found out about their pregnancies.

Invite feedback. Identify common themes.

If group members find it difficult to talk about how they feel, the educator can use prompt cards, such as those in Box 6.2, to be read out in the whole group or in small groups to stimulate discussion.

The educator needs to be aware that such an exercise may elicit strong feelings if there are people in the group seeking an opportunity to express ambivalence about their pregnancy or even hostility towards the baby. These feelings need to be acknowledged, respected and reflected back to the group to help parents explore the sources of their anger:

Box 6.2 Prompt Cards (Nolan, 1996)

Feelings about Pregnancy

'I was panic-stricken because it was completely unexpected. I had been told I probably wouldn't have children without some help and we had just a few months before started thinking about whether we ought to be on a waiting list for IVF. But we thought we'd move house first and have a good holiday and I remember telling Colin and he just sat there and said, "Well, what we are we going to do now?"'

Feelings about Pregnancy

'I was ecstatic and happy and frightened.'

Feelings about Pregnancy

'Deep down, I had desperately wanted to have a baby – there I was, pregnant!'

Feelings about Pregnancy

'We were told we were expecting twins when my partner was eight weeks pregnant and the scan showed two hearts beating. I was over the moon and immediately started speculating on what sex they would be!'

Feelings about Pregnancy

'I always used to think we'd keep it quiet for the first twelve weeks, but when it happened, we just wanted to tell everyone the minute we got that positive test.'

- 'Did anyone else feel very much in two minds about their pregnancy?'

- 'You obviously felt very strongly to begin with that you didn't want to be pregnant. How do you feel now?'

- 'Why do you think you felt so upset when you got the positive pregnancy test?'

There are a multitude of approaches that can be used to create useful opportunities for parents to consider the changes pregnancy has brought about in their lives (see Box 6.3).

Box 6.3 Changes in Pregnancy

Aim

- **to increase group members' awareness of the impact of pregnancy on self-identity and relationships**

Learning outcome

- **parents will be able to state in what ways their perception of themselves, other people's perceptions of them and their perceptions of other people have changed**

Invite class members to divide into small groups and provide each group with a different discussion prompt:

1. **How I have changed during this pregnancy.**

2. **How my partner has changed during this pregnancy.**

3. **How other people have changed towards me since I/my partner became pregnant.**

People can be asked to feed their ideas back into the large group or couples can spend a few moments sharing with each other what particularly struck them about the discussion they had in their small group.

The discussion arising from such work may include the ways in which group members' relationships with their parents have changed since finding out that they were themselves to become parents. Pregnancy may be the time when adult children reflect on their upbringing and grandparents-to-be finally recognize that their children have grown up. A baby may bring the generations closer together or may drive them apart if the parents make the decision not to involve grandparents because of memories of childhood trauma or unhappiness. Discussion in antenatal classes aims to normalize the complex emotions that pregnancy inevitably generates and to help group members consider how their own transition to parenthood forces transition on others: parents to grandparents, employers of people without parenting responsibilities to employers of people with important commitments outside work, friends of a childless couple to friends of a couple needing a babysitter before they can go out.

Helping Men Understand Their Feelings About Pregnancy

Childbirth educators have a particular responsibility to provide opportunities for men attending classes to reflect on their needs and feelings during pregnancy. As Raphael-Leff (1993) remarks:

In western societies, fathers-to-be often feel themselves to be disadvantaged ... Despite having to achieve similar changes in self-image and identity as the expectant mother, the man has no visibly growing bulge or ongoing hormonal stimulation and physical experiences of change to punctuate his paternal development. In addition, there is usually little social recognition of his transitional state. (p 158)

The educator can employ a variety of approaches to enable men to reflect on the changes that pregnancy has brought into their lives:

1. Single-sex small group work allows men to speak freely and values their experience of pregnancy equally with that of women.

2. When single-sex small groups are asked to explore the same topic and then to compare their ideas, men and women may gain greater insight into each other's fears and interpretation of events.

3. The childbirth educator can actively discriminate in favour of the men when the whole group is talking together by asking specific questions such as:

- How do you feel about the balance between home and work now that your partner is pregnant?

- Do you feel able to talk to other men about the pregnancy?

- Are there male friends with whom you can discuss what it is like to be with someone during labour and what it is like to be a father?

- How has your relationship with your own father changed during the last few months?

PARENTS AND THEIR UNBORN BABIES

The baby should be at the heart of every antenatal class. The aim of childbirth educators is to present information and to focus discussion in such a way as to enhance parents' under-standing of themselves, their baby and of their relationship with their baby. Parents-to-be whose everyday lives have never involved babies or small children need to be helped to appreciate the reality of their baby and to develop ways of thinking and being that are baby-centred. The educator can help parents to build up a picture of their baby as a unique individual already deeply engaged in a personal relationship with them. (See Box 6.4)

Childbirth educators can offer additional information about unborn babies which group members do not already know. For example, parents may be fascinated to find out that their babies already have the capacity to remember things and to learn. Such information may radically alter their perception of their baby and increase respect for him as well as deepening their relationship with a person whose 'completeness' and complexity they may not have appreciated previously. Information about the later development of the baby, such as that the sucking reflex is not established until 36 weeks' gestation and that the baby lays down reserves of fat in the last few weeks of pregnancy which he can draw on after birth whilst his mother is producing only small amounts of milk, help parents to toler-ate the final long weeks of pregnancy and understand that their baby needs to be born in his own time.

BOX 6.4 THE BABY INSIDE

Aim

- to enhance prenatal attachment between parents and their babies and so influence the quality of early parenting

Learning outcome

- group members will know what stage of development their babies have reached

Invite group members to brainstorm what their babies can do at their stage of pregnancy. The list will probably include:

- kick

- hiccough

- somersault

- wee

- hear

- see

- 'jump' when there is a sudden loud noise

Subsequent discussion can invite parents to describe their baby's pattern of waking and sleeping and how they communicate with their babies. Do they talk to their babies or sing to them?

FACILITATING LEARNING ABOUT THE BODY'S NEEDS DURING PREGNANCY

The so-called minor ailments of late pregnancy may be of little interest to health professionals, but are of immediate concern to the women who are experiencing them. If women are helped to understand the physiological basis of their discomfort, they are in a better position to cope both psychologically and practically. Whilst it is clearly not appropriate for an educator to lecture at length on the anatomy and physiology of pregnancy, people appreciate being helped to understand the relationship of the various internal organs to each other and the way in which the growing baby puts pressure on the digestive system and diaphragm. Women who are very ignorant about their own bodies are not in the best position to care for themselves or devise strategies for minimizing their discomfort. (See Box 6.5)

From this introductory exercise, it is logical to move on to practical work to help the women protect their backs and their pelvic floor muscles during late pregnancy and after the birth of their babies. (See Box 6.6)

Provided the educator is willing and confident to demonstrate the exercise and is at ease with her own body, she will probably not have any difficulty in getting the group members to

---

BOX 6.5 UNDERSTANDING HOW PREGNANCY AFFECTS THE MOTHER'S BODY

Aim

- to increase each woman's understanding and awareness of her own body

Learning outcome

- group members will know some of the ways in which the woman's anatomy and physiology are affected by pregnancy

Using a large cross-sectional picture of the pregnant female body, invite class members to name the various organs. Or prepare labels with 'uterus', 'placenta', 'umbilical cord', 'back passage', 'bladder', 'urethra', 'vagina', 'intestines', 'lungs', 'diaphragm' written on them and invite class members to Blu-tak the labels on to the chart.

(This exercise might not be suitable for antenatal groups which include people from certain ethnic minority groups who consider naming the sexual parts of the woman's body offensive (Schott and Henley, 1996, p 158).)

Using a variety of questions, invite class members to consider how pregnancy might affect a woman's body:

- What parts of the body do you think the weight of the baby will put particular strain upon?

- What aches and pains have the women in the group experienced which this chart could explain? How are you coping with them?

---

practise the exercise with her. If the educator is ill at ease, it is unlikely that class members will benefit from the learning opportunity she is trying to provide.

Childbirth educators who subscribe to the theory of optimal fetal positioning (Sutton, 1996) may wish to help mothers understand how sitting with their knees lower than their hips from 35 weeks of pregnancy and crawling on their hands and knees for a period each day encourage babies to enter the pelvis in the anterior position. Educators who are seeing women on a regular basis at the very end of their pregnancies are in an excellent position to remind them of the best way to sit.

Childbirth educators are often worried about teaching pelvic floor muscle exercises to mixed groups. Difficulties centre around the feeling that these exercises are not relevant to male class attenders and may cause embarrassment. Educators who feel strongly that pelvic floor exercises should be taught to everyone attending their classes argue that men need to exercise their pelvic floor muscles in order to avoid prostate problems in later life, that, if men understand the importance of the exercises to their partners' health, they will encourage the women to practise, and that it is divisive in antenatal classes to exclude men from some activities.

Some mixed groups will respond in a very relaxed manner to learning pelvic floor exercises; others comprised of people who have not settled down well together, or which include individuals who are very shy, may not find a mixed group an appropriate learning

BOX 6.6 PROTECTING YOUR BACK

Aim

- to minimize the risk of long-term back problems stemming from pregnancy

Learning outcome

- group members will be able to state the importance of and adopt a good posture in late pregnancy

Invite each woman to stand with her back against a wall, bending her knees slightly so that her shoulder blades and bottom are touching the wall. Ask her to rock her pelvis forwards so that the hollow in her back flattens against the wall. To test that she has carried out the exercise correctly, invite her partner or supporter to slip their hand in the hollow of her back and to tell her whether they can feel her back flattening against their hand as she rocks her pelvis forward.
(Male partners and non-pregnant women in the group can also try the exercise with the pregnant women giving feedback.)

When everyone feels confident that they know how to do the movement, ask the group members to stand clear of the wall, and with their knees straight (but not locked) to rock their pelvises forwards so that the hollow in their backs becomes flatter. Remind the group to breathe as they are doing the exercise. Explain that this posture protects the natural 'S' bend of the spine from becoming overstrained, resulting in chronic low back pain.

BOX 6.7 IDENTIFYING PELVIC FLOOR MUSCLES

Aim

- to promote short- and long-term health of the pelvic floor muscles

Learning outcome

- class attenders will be able to identify their pelvic floor muscles

Invite class members to place their clenched fists over their mouths. If they now cough into their fists, they should feel their pelvic floor muscles bulging between their legs.

Demonstrate with a model pelvis where the pelvic floor muscles are sited.

Invite class members to imagine a situation where they need to use the toilet but it is already occupied. The muscles that they use 'to hang on' are their pelvic floor muscles.

environment for this kind of practical work. If the educator herself is unsure about how to include the men, she might be better to teach the exercises in a single-sex group until she has had the time to talk to other antenatal educators about her feelings, share experiences, and discuss a variety of teaching approaches.

Neither women nor men will be likely to persist on a daily basis in exercising their pelvic floors unless they have a clear understanding of the reasons why they need to. Before she can start to teach any exercises, the educator must ensure that class attenders understand the short- and long-term benefits of maintaining pelvic floor muscle function and help class members identify the muscles in question. (See Box 6.7)

It is easier for people to learn to exercise their pelvic floor muscles in a standing position, leaning forwards on to the back of a chair or table. This position makes the sensations of

---

BOX 6.8 TEACHING PELVIC FLOOR MUSCLE EXERCISES

Aim

- to promote short- and long-term health of the pelvic floor muscles

Learning outcome

- class attenders will have developed the skill of exercising the different fibres that comprise their pelvic floor muscles

Invite group members to tighten the muscles around their back passage and then the muscles around the vagina or penis as if they are trying to avoid passing wind. Then ask the group to tighten their muscles more and more, imagining that they have a lift between their legs and are taking the lift up to the first floor, then the second and then the third.

Remind the group to continue to breathe whilst doing the exercise.

After pausing on the top floor, invite the group members to relax their muscles a little down to the second floor, then a little more down to the first floor and finally, to relax them fully as they come down to the ground floor.

After a pause, invite the group to push their muscles out as if going down to the basement.

Explain that, when they are giving birth to their babies, the women will need to let their pelvic floor muscles 'bulge' as if they were doing the 'basement' part of the exercise.

Invite the group members to take a few deep breaths, letting their shoulders drop and relaxing on the out-breath, before asking them to exercise the 'flick' fibres of their pelvic floor muscles.

Invite them to tighten their pelvic floor muscles as firmly as they can, holding for a count of one, and then to relax the muscles for a count of one. Ask them to repeat this pattern of tightening and relaxing ten times whilst counting out loud: 1 – 2 – 1 – 2 – 1 – 2 – 1 – 2 – 1 – 2 – 1 – 2 – 1 – 2 – 1 – 2 – 1 – 2 – 1 – 2.

tightening and then relaxing the muscles more acute and gives a greater sense of achievement when practising. (See Box 6.8)

There seems to be a lot of conflicting advice about how often women should exercise their pelvic floor muscles. It is probably not helpful to tell women that they should practise 100 times a day; most people will respond to such a demand by doing nothing at all. It may be more useful to brainstorm with group members how they can remember to exercise regularly each day. Suggestions might include:

1. Exercising at fixed times each day, for example:

- first thing in the morning, and

- during the lunch break, and

- last thing at night

2. Associating pelvic floor muscle exercises with an activity that is carried out several times a day:

- picking up toys

- stopping at red traffic lights

- washing up

- having a cup of coffee

HELPING CLASS MEMBERS LEARN ABOUT PRE-ECLAMPSIA

Women and their partners are empowered to participate in decision-making when they are familiar with the terminology used by midwives and doctors and understand the particular indicators that their carers use to assess well-being during pregnancy. It is therefore important for the childbirth educator to discuss the hand-held notes that each woman carries, asking whether people understand the abbreviations used and the significance of the examinations the women have during their clinic visits. Helping parents understand the warning signs of pre-eclampsia is an essential part of such a discussion. The childbirth educator needs to find out what they already know so that she is in a position to correct any misconceptions:

- 'Do you know of anyone who has suffered from pre-eclampsia? What happened?'

- 'What have you already heard about pre-eclampsia?'

She is responsible for ensuring that each woman knows the circumstances under which she should consult her midwife or doctor. Whilst it is important not to scaremonger, it is also vital to ensure that this information has been received and that it is consolidated at the end of the session or at a later session.

TEACHING QUESTION-ASKING SKILLS

Pregnancy is a time when people seek information; they have, perhaps, a greater thirst for and need of information than at any other time in their lives. Information puts parents in a position to share in decision-making about their care and to grow in confidence that they can give birth to their baby and be 'good-enough' parents. One of the ways in which women and their supporters can be empowered to obtain the information they need is by attending classes with a childbirth educator who encourages questions and is open to all their ideas. The willingness of the childbirth educator to listen to their questions, to provide full and balanced information and to invite their opinions will encourage them to insist on similar communication from those who care for them during labour and after the birth.

Teaching parents how to communicate effectively helps them to be in control of their labour. Research suggests that women want to be consulted about and share in the ordinary decisions that need to be made during childbirth:

- 'Most women wanted at least to have non-emergency decisions discussed with them and to be in control of what staff did to them.'

- 'The majority of women wanted to know as much as possible about what might happen in labour.' (Green et al, 1988, Chapter 4)

Exercises that enable class members to acquire question-asking skills are a useful part of antenatal classes. (See Box 6.9)

The childbirth educator can use such an exercise to help class members look at the differences between passive, aggressive and assertive communication; to explore the different

---

BOX 6.9 QUESTION-ASKING SKILLS

Aim

- **to enable women and their supporters to make informed choices**

Learning outcome

- **class members will have developed skills to enable them to obtain the information they need from their carers**

Invite class members to participate in an easy role play. Reassure them that their lines are already written for them.

Explain that the role plays describe three encounters between a couple and their carers. The woman is in strong labour, but her cervix is not dilating very quickly. Her doctor suggests breaking the waters.

Ask the class members not involved in the role play to listen carefully to how the father obtains information.

Scene 1
Characters: doctor, father, mother

Doctor:	**Your labour is progressing very slowly. I think we ought to break your waters.**
Father:	**Oh dear. Do you think that's OK, darling?**
Mother:	**I don't know.**
Father:	**Well, if that's what you're advising, doctor, we'll go along with you.**
Doctor:	**Fine. It will only take a few minutes to organise.**

Scene 2

Characters: doctor, father, mother

Doctor: Your labour is progressing very slowly. I think we ought to break your waters.

(The father responds angrily; he stands up and puts his face very close to the doctor's.)

Father: Definitely not! We're doing fine and we don't want any interference. The baby's not in distress, is it?

Doctor: Well, no, but . . .

Father: So! There's nothing to talk about.

(The doctor sighs heavily and walks out.)

Scene 3

Characters: doctor, father, mother, midwife

Doctor: Your labour is progressing very slowly. I think we ought to break your waters.

Father: Right! Can I just ask you a few questions so that we can make up our minds. Is this an emergency situation?

Doctor: No. But labour is very slow. The baby's fine and your partner's coping well.

Father: So why do we need to do anything?

Doctor: If we break the waters, it might speed labour up a bit and that means that your partner and the baby won't get exhausted.

Father: Are there any risks involved?

Doctor: A few. The contractions could become much stronger, so your partner might want to have some pethidine or an epidural. Most people have no problems after the waters have been broken, but some do find the change in pace difficult. The baby might become distressed if the labour suddenly gets stronger. There is also a slight risk of infection.

Midwife
(to mother):   We could try some different positions to see whether that helps speed things up. Why don't you stand up for a little while and walk around in between contractions?

Father: Can we talk about breaking the waters in another hour or so?

Doctor: OK. Let's wait a little longer and see what happens. Is that your decision?

Mother: Yes.

Doctor: Fine.

After each role play, invite class members to discuss what happened and whether they consider they would be likely to react as the father did in similar encounters with health professionals.

roles of doctor and midwife; to think about emergency and non-emergency decision-making; and, coincidentally, to learn about artificial rupture of membranes.

CONCLUSION

Traditionally, although not necessarily ideally, parents and their supporters attend antenatal classes in late pregnancy. Information-sharing and discussion about pregnancy may not seem very relevant to them when their agenda for classes is often focused exclusively on labour and the early weeks of parenting. However, it is important for the childbirth educator to help clients understand that labour is merely a part of the ongoing transition to parenthood that started at conception and is in a critical phase during pregnancy. Parents' ability to engage in a relationship with their unborn babies and to prepare themselves for parenting will be enhanced when their antenatal classes include a focus on the complex physical and emotional adjustments that pregnancy involves. Question-asking skills are vital if parents want to be informed consumers of the maternity services and maintain control over their own care.

KEY POINTS

1. Antenatal education provides parents with an opportunity to explore their reactions to their pregnancy, their feelings about their unborn child, and changes in their relationships with others and in their perceptions of themselves.

2. The childbirth educator aims to help pregnant parents who have no experience of babies to appreciate the reality of their baby and to develop ways of thinking and being that are baby-centred.

3. Acquiring question-asking skills enables clients to participate more fully in decision-making during labour and early parenting.

REFERENCES

Antonucci TC and Mikus K (1988) Personality and attitudinal changes. In Michaels GY and Goldberg WA (eds) *The Transition to Parenthood: Current Theory and Research*, pp 62–84. Cambridge: Cambridge University Press.

Green J, Coupland V and Kitzinger J (1988) *Great Expectations: A Prospective Study of Women's Expectations and Experiences of Childbirth*, Vol. 1. University of Cambridge: Child Care and Development Group.

Nolan M (1996) *Being Pregnant, Giving Birth*, pp 1, 3. Cambridge: National Childbirth Trust in association with HMSO.

Raphael-Leff J (1993) *Psychological Processes of Childbearing*. London: Chapman and Hall.

Schott J and Henley A (1996) *Culture, Religion and Childbearing in Multiracial Britain*. Oxford: Butterworth–Heinemann.

Sutton J (1996) *Understanding and Teaching Optimal Foetal Positioning*. Tauranga, New Zealand: Birth Concepts.

Practical Skills Work
for Labour

7

PERCEPTIONS OF PAIN

Although many women attend aerobics classes, work out in the gym regularly or participate in a sport, they can be surprisingly ignorant about how their bodies work. Women from the technologically advanced countries of the world are often out of touch with their reproductive cycles, which are controlled for them by the contraceptive pill, and lack confidence in helping themselves cope with pain and illness. The body may be seen by women (and men) as something to be subjugated rather than to be worked with. When they come to give birth, women may find themselves doubly disadvantaged, firstly by their lack of understanding of their own bodies, and secondly by conflicting thinking about pain.

Pain is generally seen in Western societies as undesirable and demeaning (Eggers, 1995). Advances in medicine throughout the twentieth century mean that people's experience of pain during their lives has been greatly reduced. None the less, the availability of epidurals – which offer the possibility, if not the certainty, of pain-free childbirth – remains problematical for many women. Today, the primary concern of women who expect to have only a few pregnancies during their reproductive years is that their babies enjoy optimum conditions in the womb, during birth and in the early days of life. As medical knowledge has become more widely available to a better educated public, and consumer groups have pointed out some of the possible dangers of drug use during childbirth, women have found themselves increasingly torn between a mistrust of pain which is part of their social consciousness and a new awareness of the possible side-effects of interventions in labour. The medical profession also finds itself divided between practitioners who consider it an essential part of their vocation to relieve pain and those who make a distinction between pathological and physiological pain:

> One perspective on obstetric anesthesia can be summarized by the following quotation: 'Labor results in severe pain for many women. There is no other circumstance where it is considered acceptable for a person to experience severe pain, amenable to safe intervention,

while under a physician's care. Maternal request is sufficient justification for pain relief in labor.' However, many health care workers and consumers point out that labor pain is physiologic, has never caused morbidity or mortality, and therefore should not be treated as if it is pathologic. Death and permanent morbidity are attendant risks, albeit small, of epidural analgesia. This viewpoint is eloquently stated by one anesthesiologist: 'The practice of obstetric anesthesia is unique in medicine in that we use an invasive and potentially hazardous procedure to provide a humanitarian service to healthy women undergoing a physiological process'. (Thorp and Breedlove, 1996, p 81)

When asked to draw up a list of the topics they want to cover during their antenatal classes, women commonly put 'coping with pain' at the top. Many would like to go through labour without any form of medical pain relief, but are doubtful of their ability to cope. This attitude exactly mirrors their feelings about breastfeeding; many would like to 'try' to breastfeed their babies, but buy sterilizing equipment 'just in case'. There is a crisis of confidence in the natural functioning of the body, whether it be to control the pain of childbirth or to provide sufficient milk for a new baby.

Childbirth for women who are the well nourished and healthy daughters and granddaughters of women who also enjoyed the advantages of good living conditions and easy access to health care has never been safer. The finely adjusted mechanics of birth have never been more likely to prove themselves equal to the task of bringing a baby into the world. The aim of antenatal education must therefore be to empower women to trust in their bodies and in their natural ability to give birth to their babies:

I want to give women confidence in their own bodies, confidence in what their bodies can actually achieve because it's the woman's body that's delivering this baby, not the midwife. (Parentcraft Sister, 1995)

My aim is to give women a practical experience of their own bodies and to show them how to use their bodies in labour because it's the body that has to give birth – there isn't a brain cell in your head during labour, is there?! (Active Birth Teacher, 1995)

The philosophy of contemporary health care is that the client has the right to make her own choices about the care she receives. Antenatal education, therefore, has a responsibility to enable women to choose a non-medicated delivery as well as informing them about the types of medical pain relief available to them. Women who have little knowledge of or trust in their bodies need to be shown how they can help themselves during labour if they want to choose natural forms of pain control. At present, many women coming to antenatal classes are not in a position to make a choice about pain relief because they are ignorant of their own resources for coping with pain and of how these can enable the mechanics of labour to work more smoothly.

PROVIDING A RATIONALE FOR PRACTICAL SKILLS WORK

Women cannot learn to work with their bodies by sitting around in discussion groups. If they are to acquire confidence in the skills that will help them cope with labour, they must practise them on a regular basis. To overcome the reluctance that many people may feel to join in practical skills work, the educator needs to provide an underpinning rationale that is both convincing and empowering.

The ways in which individuals cope with pain may be very different and it is the educator's aim to enable each woman in her class to draw on her own unique coping strategies. Adult learners are able to refer to previous experiences of pain in order to inform their thinking about coping with pain in labour (Yerby, 1996). A discussion that enables people to understand their own coping mechanisms may be initiated with a question such as:

'If you think back to a time when you had a painful illness or injury, what sort of things helped you cope?'

Class members may mention:

- making a lot of noise

- using hot water bottles or ice packs

- having other people offer support and reassurance

- rubbing the injured part

- lying down and curling up

- darkness

- seeing a doctor or nurse

- being told the extent of the injury or how long the illness would last

- taking pain killers

The educator can show how all of these might apply in labour and point out that the use of drugs to control pain is only one strategy amongst the many with which the group is already familiar.

Group members' perceptions of labour pain may change if the educator invites them to consider how the pain of labour is different from that of illness or injury, and helps them understand that, while pain normally indicates that the body is damaged, labour pain indicates that the body is functioning healthily. The educator can explain that the pain of labour:

1. enables the woman to know when her labour has started so that she can choose a safe place (home or hospital) for her baby to be born and summon people to help her (her labour supporter(s) and midwife).

2. enables the woman to know how far on in labour she is; as the contractions become stronger and more frequent, the woman knows that the time for her baby to be born is getting closer.

3. tells the woman what she should do to help her baby be born more easily. The woman responds to her contractions by trying to find comfortable positions to ease her pain; by moving around, regularly changing her position, she encourages the cervix to dilate evenly and helps her baby make the necessary moves through the pelvis.

4. directs the woman when and how to push in second stage. Women who are not directed how to push in second stage give birth more quickly and to healthier babies than women who are told when they should push and for how long (Caldeyro-Barcia, 1979)

It often comes as a revelation to women that they may be able to work with their contractions to maintain control over their labour and assist the birth of their babies.

When introducing practical skills work in classes, the educator needs to:

- explain clearly what it is that group members are being asked to do

- offer verbal and physical support to individuals while they are practising

- stress the benefits that class members will derive from practising these skills

If the antenatal course consists of a series of classes, practical skills work can be started at the first session so that, right from the beginning, the model is being drawn that labour is not a cerebral activity but an intensely physical one. The longer practical skills work is delayed, the harder it will be for the childbirth educator to get people to participate.

TEACHING PHYSICAL SKILLS FOR LABOUR

If a childbirth educator is to be successful in facilitating practical skills work for labour in her classes, it is essential that she has a firm belief in the ability of most women to give birth to their babies without intervention and in the efficacy of natural forms of pain relief to assist the birth process. Unless the educator is convinced that women have resources which, in a favourable environment, can enable them to give birth without medical assistance, she is unlikely to convince class members that learning about those resources will be of service to them.

Even if the environment of hospital birth is likely to make it difficult for women to use to the full the skills they have learnt during their antenatal classes (because the delivery rooms are small, clinical and dominated by a bed; because of lack of privacy; because women in hospital feel that they are guests in someone else's workplace; because they are constantly reminded that there is a 24-hour-a-day epidural service available), there is still a case to be made for helping them learn some natural pain control mechanisms. First, childbirth educators need to transmit their belief in the strength and resourcefulness of women's bodies during labour as a way of protecting women's understanding of and trust in themselves. Second, educators should remember that the skills taught to a primiparous woman may not bear fruit during her first labour, but may well do so during her second or third. Many women find that, when they have their second babies, they are more relaxed and more confident in utilizing their own resources. The skills they learned when they were first pregnant then come into their own.

Childbirth educators will hear lots of women talking postnatally about how marvellous their epidural was or how thankful they were for the rest that a shot of pethidine gave them during the most difficult part of their labour. It is easy to tune into such comments and feel that there is no point in practising self-help skills during antenatal classes. However, there are other stories being told, even if not so commonly:

I tried to relax during the contractions and I took my walkman and we'd taped my favourite songs and I listened to them over and over again and that helped me relax.

When I was having contractions, I needed to hold someone's hand. Gas and air was offered to me, but I grabbed somebody's hand rather than gas and air. That got me over it.

What really helped me was the massage – I wanted more, harder, harder. It was wonderful. I suppose it added pressure but was taking it away at the same time. It was brilliant. (Nolan, 1996; pp 101, 102, 104)

RELAXATION: INTRODUCING THE CONCEPT

It is established in the literature (Strychar et al, 1990) that women are especially open to making changes in their lives during pregnancy. If women are given a full explanation, in language that they can understand, of the benefits for them and their babies of changing their lifestyles, they will often respond very positively. Many women are persuaded to give up smoking or reduce the number of cigarettes they smoke while they are pregnant. Some will never smoke again. Whilst advice on improving eating habits and smoking cessation is best given either pre-conception or in early pregnancy, the childbirth educator, who may not meet her clients until much later, still has a wonderful opportunity to help women and their partners acquire relaxation skills. Today's childbearing women, born and brought up in the post Dick-Read era, generally expect that their antenatal classes will include 'relaxation' and 'breathing', and are open to what the educator has to say.

People do not need to be told about the benefits of relaxation; they already know, even if they have not consciously thought about them and even if they do not include opportunities to relax in their lives. A brainstorming session starting with an open-ended question:

How do you feel when you are relaxed?

will elicit nearly all the points the childbirth educator might want to make on the subject:

- I feel happy/confident.
- I can enjoy myself.
- I feel full of energy.
- I can stop worrying about work.
- I feel I can cope.
- I can get things in proportion.

All these points can be related to the labour situation, enabling class members to appreciate how relaxing during labour will empower them to cope better, conserve their energy, be less frightened, communicate more effectively and enjoy the birth of their babies more.

Class members may need to broaden their understanding of the factors that will influence their ability to relax during labour. Many people's ideas about relaxation centre on visualization, or mantras, or stretching and relaxing exercises. These are specific techniques that can help women (and their supporters) relax during labour, but the childbirth educator needs to help her group consider all the other issues that influence relaxation. (See Boxes 7.1, 7.2 and Fig. 7.1)

The childbirth educator can use an exercise like this to help class members understand that there are things they can do before labour starts – such as getting information about the hospital, choosing a supportive companion and preparing a birth plan – as well as during labour, which will help them to feel relaxed.

Many people today lead extremely busy lives and have little experience of how their bodies feel when truly relaxed. To introduce class members to relaxation, it is helpful to start with simple exercises which point out the contrast between stretched and relaxed muscles. The first session of an antenatal course might usefully include an exercise in progressive muscular relaxation. (See Box 7.3)

If the childbirth educator is new to leading relaxation sessions, it is very helpful, and probably essential, for her to practise with her partner, friends or colleagues beforehand and to ask for detailed feedback, especially about the way she *paces* the exercise. The temptation is always to go through a sequence such as the one outlined above far too quickly. Pauses seem much longer to the person leading the relaxation session than to those participating in it, but people need plenty of time to respond to one suggestion before they can listen to another.

Box 7.1 Introducing Relaxation

Aim

- to raise group members' awareness of the part played by stress and relaxation in their daily lives

Learning outcomes

Group members will be able to:

- state how stress affects them

- describe a range of everyday relaxation techniques

- adapt everyday relaxation techniques to labour

Ask for a volunteer to lie on three pieces of flipchart paper taped together and placed on the floor. (Explain that s/he is going to provide the outline of a person.)

Give marker pens to some of the group and ask them to draw round the volunteer.

When the outline is finished, the volunteer can get up and group members be asked to indicate with arrows or drawings all the parts of the body that are affected by stress.

At the top of the sheet, ask people to write down some of the causes of stress in their lives.
At the bottom of the sheet, ask people to write down the things that help them to relax.

Discuss the effects of tension: how a little adrenaline helps people to perform at their best, but too much is counterproductive. Relate stress to labour and discuss its effects on mother and baby.

Ask people to say how they could apply their daily relaxation strategies to labour.

At the end of the relaxation sequence, the educator needs to ask class members for feedback. Did they enjoy the session? Do they feel relaxed now? How did the babies respond while the women were relaxing? When the mother is deeply relaxed, oxygen supplies to her baby are abundant and the baby has lots of energy for kicking. Women can thus link their physical and mental state with a particular response from their babies.

While it is important that parents gain an understanding of how to relax in a calm environment when they have time to concentrate on each part of their body in turn, education about relaxation needs to be made relevant to the labour situation and to the demands of caring for tiny babies and demanding toddlers, children or teenagers. Class members can try out a variety of techniques to help them cope with stressful situations when there are only a few seconds or minutes available for relaxing. (See Box 7.4)

98

BOX 7.2 ABOUT RELAXATION

Aim

- to raise class members' awareness of the many factors that affect relaxation during labour

Learning outcomes

Class members will be able to:

- describe the preparations they can make to help themselves relax during labour
- communicate with and obtain information from their carers during labour

Invite group members to think of a time when they had to face a stressful situation such as:

- going for an interview
- having major dental work
- taking part in a marathon

Ask

- How did you prepare yourself beforehand?
- What things helped you relax while the event was taking place?

Write associated ideas on a flipchart in clusters around the keyword 'Relaxation'; for example:

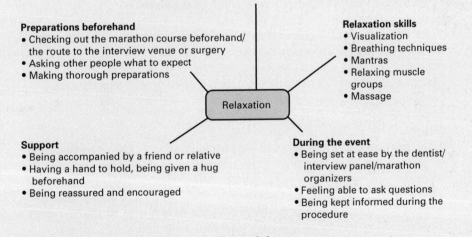

On the day
- Having something to eat/drink beforehand
- Wearing the right clothes
- Having the right equipment/comfort aids to hand
- Comfortable environment at the surgery/interview venue

Preparations beforehand
- Checking out the marathon course beforehand/ the route to the interview venue or surgery
- Asking other people what to expect
- Making thorough preparations

Relaxation skills
- Visualization
- Breathing techniques
- Mantras
- Relaxing muscle groups
- Massage

Relaxation

Support
- Being accompanied by a friend or relative
- Having a hand to hold, being given a hug beforehand
- Being reassured and encouraged

During the event
- Being set at ease by the dentist/ interview panel/marathon organizers
- Feeling able to ask questions
- Being kept informed during the procedure

Go through the lists and apply each idea to labour

BOX 7.3 PROGRESSIVE MUSCULAR RELAXATION

Aim

- to increase class members' awareness of their own bodies

Learning outcome

- class members will be able to achieve whole body relaxation

Acknowledge that it is difficult to relax in a room full of people (although this may be the situation during labour.) Invite class members to join in the relaxation session as fully as possible. Give permission for people not to participate if they choose, but ask them to keep their eyes lowered so as not to distract others.

Dim the lights (if possible), explaining that bright lights stimulate the talking, doing, active centres of the brain, and invite people to make themselves as comfortable as possible in their chairs or on the floor.

Speaking gently but clearly, lead the group through a short relaxation sequence:

> *Close your eyes if that helps you relax. If you don't want to, keep your eyes open but lowered so that you don't distract anyone else.*
> *Listen to your own breathing. Notice how the in-breath balances the out-breath. Notice how rhythmical your breathing is.*
> *(Pause)*
> *Now I'm going to ask you to stretch various muscles in your body and then relax them.*
> *Start with your feet. Curl your toes gently – and then let them relax.*
> *(Pause)*
> *Tighten your thigh muscles – and then let them relax.*
> *Feel how heavy your legs are now.*
> *(Pause)*
> *Tighten your tummy muscles – now relax your tummy.*
> *(Pause)*
> *Make fists with your hands and feel the tension – now relax your hands so that your fingers are softly curled.*
> *(Pause)*
> *Pull your shoulders up towards your ears. Notice how that makes your breathing tight and uncomfortable. Relax your shoulders and breathe freely again.*
> *(Pause)*
> *Now frown as angrily as you can, screwing up all your face muscles. Now let the tension go so that there is no expression at all on your face.*
> *(Pause)*
> *Take a moment to check that your whole body is relaxed. Your forehead is smooth and tall. Your jaw is relaxed – your mouth may be slightly open. Your shoulders feel loose and easy, and your arms and hands are soft*

and relaxed. Your tummy is relaxed. Your legs and feet are heavy. You feel
warm and peaceful.
(Pause)
While you are relaxed, take a moment to think about your baby. How
warm and safe she or he is in the womb. How much you are looking
forward to meeting your baby.
(Pause)
Now I'm going to count from 5 down to 1. Use that time to stretch,
yawn, open your eyes and sit up straight again.
5 – 4 – 3 – 2 – 1.

BOX 7.4 QUICK RELAXATIONS

Aim

- to increase class members' confidence in their ability to relax in between contractions or in stressful life situations

Learning outcome

- class members will be able to achieve a relaxed state in a few moments

Exercise 1

Explain to class members that this exercise is designed to help them relax in stressful situations such as when contractions are coming at very short intervals or when they feel at the end of their tether with a crying baby.

Ask everyone to stand and take a deep breath in, then to sigh their breath out and, as they breathe out, to imagine their breath carrying away tension from their shoulders, hands, tummy and legs. Remind people not to *force* their breath out, but to let it *flow* out. Suggest that the lungs will fill again of their own accord when they are ready.
Repeat the exercise.

Exercise 2

Write on a flipchart five words beginning with 'S' associated with relaxation:

| SHAKE | SWING | STROKE | STRETCH | SMILE |

1. Invite people to stand and SHAKE out their hands gently.

2. Invite them to hold on to the back of a chair and shake each foot in turn.

3. Next SWING their arms first to the right and then to the left, twisting their bodies but keeping their feet stationary.

4. Ask them to STROKE their foreheads from the bridge of the nose out to the temples.

5. Then to stand and STRETCH upwards with their arms and hands reaching into the air and rising on to their tiptoes if they want to.

6. Finally, ask them to SMILE, suggesting that it is hard to be tense and bad-tempered if you are smiling with a soft, relaxed smile.

Exercise 3

Explain to class members that women in labour need to have physical contact with those who are supporting them and that this exercise is one way of using touch to help someone relax.

Ask everyone to stand up and the women to stand with their backs towards their supporters. Invite each supporter to place his/her hands on top of the mother's head and to stroke gently but firmly down the side of her face, over her shoulders, down her arms and off at her finger tips. Then to place his/her hands on top of the mother's shoulders and stroke down each side of her spine, down the backs of her legs and off at her toes.

Invite people working together to swap over so that everyone has the chance to experience the relaxing effect of being stroked.

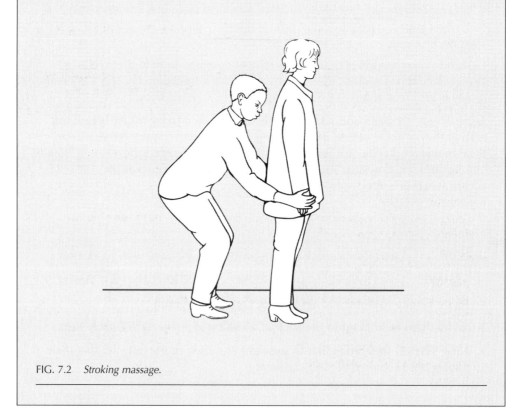

FIG. 7.2 *Stroking massage.*

The relevance of these exercises can be reinforced by asking class members to think of situations in which the ability to relax quickly might be useful, such as when a quarrel is about to break out; when the toddler has drawn on the wallpaper; when the health visitor arrives just as the baby has dropped off to sleep . . .

TEACHING BREATHING PATTERNS FOR LABOUR

Breathing is one of the fundamental rhythms of life. In stressful situations, such as labour, the rhythm may be disrupted and hyperventilation may occur, with ill-effects for baby and mother. When parents learn in their antenatal classes how to achieve a relaxed state through their breathing, they have acquired a skill that will stand them in good stead for the rest of their lives. The first step towards using breathing patterns as a pain-control technique in labour is for people to become aware of the rhythm of their own breathing. (See Box 7.5)

There is still much debate amongst childbirth educators about the value of teaching breathing patterns for labour. Although the Lamaze method of childbirth preparation, which

---

BOX 7.5 BREATHING AND RELAXATION

Aim

- **to increase parents' and supporters' understanding of the link between breathing and relaxation**

Learning outcome

- **Parents and supporters will be able to use the rhythm of their breathing to help them relax**

Invite people to participate in a relaxation session which focuses specifically on breathing patterns. Ask whether it is all right to dim the lights to make the environment more private and relaxing.

Talk through the following sequence:

Make sure you're quite comfortable. If at any time you become uncomfortable, feel free to change your position so that you're comfortable again.
(Pause)
Listen now to your own breathing. Notice the balance between your in-breath and your out-breath.
(Pause)
Your in-breath and your out-breath.
(Pause)
Each time you breathe out, drop your shoulders and relax.
(Pause)
Let the air fill your lungs when you are ready to breathe in. Don't suck the breath in. Just let it flow in.
And relax on the out-breath.
(Pause)

So each time you breathe out, you're feeling a little more relaxed, a little heavier and warmer.

(Pause)

Now I'm going to ask you to imagine that you're breathing in through and out of various parts of your body. As you breathe out, relax that part of your body.

Start with your right leg. Imagine that you're breathing in through your right leg (Pause) and out through it, and relax it on the out-breath.

(Pause)

Now your left leg. Breathe in through it (Pause) and out through it, and relax it on the out-breath.

(Pause)

Now your tummy. Imagine that you're breathing in through it (Pause) and out through it and relax it on the out-breath.

(Pause)

Now your right arm and hand. Imagine that you're breathing in through them (Pause) and out through them, and relax them on the out-breath.

(Pause)

Now your left arm and hand. Imagine that you're breathing in through them (Pause) and out through them, and relax them on the out-breath.

(Pause)

Breathe in through your shoulders (Pause) and out through them, and relax them on the out-breath.

(Pause)

And finally, your head. Breathe in through your head (Pause) and out through it, and relax it on the out-breath.

(Pause)

Spend a few moments concentrating on your breathing and thinking to yourself 're' as you breathe in and 'lax' as you breathe out and relax.

(Pause)

When you are ready, gently move and open your eyes and sit up.

When everyone is alert again, ask for feedback:

- Did you enjoy the exercise?

- How did it make you feel?

- What did you notice about your breathing as we went through the exercise?

has for many years been the cornerstone of antenatal classes, especially in the United States, places great emphasis on coaching women and their partners in breathing techniques, the fashion for teaching 'levels of breathing' has fallen out of favour in the UK. Childbirth educators have become concerned that women whose preparation for labour focuses almost exclusively on breathing patterns are especially vulnerable to a sense of failure if they find that what they have learned is insufficient to help them cope with the pain of strong contractions. There are women who find that breathing very shallowly over the top of a contraction as taught by some

Lamaze instructors tends to precipitate hyperventilation; others simply forget all they have learned as soon as labour starts.

There are childbirth educators who are uneasy about imposing in any way on the woman's instinctive response to contractions and decide that, rather than teaching breathing techniques, it is better to encourage her to listen to what her body tells her to do during labour. Those who continue to teach 'breathing for labour' (of whom the present author is one) hope to give women a tool for coping with the pain of contractions and, by making them aware of the problem of hyperventilation, help them to avoid it. The emphasis is very much on helping the woman learn how to keep her breathing rhythmical. This rhythm is achieved in labour by focusing on the *out-breath* because in situations of great stress or panic, it is the out-breath that is either held back or shortened, so giving rise to the classical symptoms of hyperventilation – light-headedness, pins and needles, and clawing of the hands.

Helping women and their supporters to understand hyperventilation is a vital component of the health promotional aspect of antenatal classes. People who know how to help themselves cope with panic retain control of the situation when they would otherwise become dependent on others. Knowing how to help another person, perhaps a child, who is panicking is a useful skill in a crisis.

A good way to start class attenders thinking about breathing is to help them understand where exactly their lungs are and how versatile their breathing is. (See Box 7.6)

Following on from this exercise, the educator can ask group members to consider what happens to their breathing when they are frightened or in pain. If their breathing becomes shallow and tight, how does that make them feel? The points to lead on to are:

BOX 7.6 UNDERSTANDING BREATHING PATTERNS

Aim

- to increase class attenders' awareness of the physiological process of breathing

Learning outcome

- class attenders will be able to identify the apex and base of their lungs and to demonstrate shallow and deep breathing

Invite people to work in couples/pairs with the pregnant woman sitting sideways on a chair. Her partner places his hands on her waist and asks her to breathe deeply into his hands. He next moves his hands to the middle of the woman's back and she breathes at that level. Finally, he moves his hands to just below her shoulders and the woman breathes very shallowly into his hands.

The childbirth educator can draw the following points from this exercise:

1. that the lungs take up a considerable amount of space in the body

2. that we often do not use them to their full capacity

3. that breathing is essentially rhythmical. No matter how deep or how shallow, it is comfortable only when the in-breath is evenly matched by the out-breath.

- that it is natural for people to breathe more shallowly when they are in a stressful situation such as labour

- that this is all right as long as the breathing remains rhythmical with the out-breath balancing the in-breath

- that the out-breath can be held back when people are very stressed and that it is important to focus on breathing *out* during labour. The in-breath will take care of itself.

There are a number of ways in which women can be helped to maintain a good breathing rhythm in labour. Practising a variety of techniques during classes gives people confidence that they will be able to help themselves in labour. (See Box 7.7)

BOX 7.7 BREATHING TECHNIQUES

Aim

- **to boost the confidence of women and their supporters that they have in-built resources for coping with stress and pain**

Learning outcome

- **class attenders will have acquired breathing skills that emphasize the importance of the out-breath balancing the in-breath**

Technique 1
Invite class attenders to shut their eyes and to breathe in through their noses and blow out gently through their mouths. Remind them not to force the out-breath out, but to blow gently until they feel that their lungs want to fill again. Ask them to focus on breathing in this way for half a minute or so, dropping their shoulders each time they breathe out.

Technique 2
Invite class members to shut their eyes and breathe in to a count of three and out to a count of three. If this number is not comfortable for them, invite them to choose another number which better represents the length of their in- and out-breaths. Remind people to drop their shoulders each time they breathe out.

Technique 3
Invite class members to shut their eyes and breathe in easily. As they breathe out, ask them to say quietly 'o-u-t', and to relax and drop their shoulders.

It is useful for labour supporters to consider ways in which to help a woman whose breathing becomes panicky during labour. It is possible that there are people in the class who have helped others through panic attacks or had to cope with them themselves. A brain-storming session drawing on these experiences will highlight the need to support the person who is panicking by:

- close physical contact

- reassurance

- eye contact

- practical assistance

The childbirth educator can then invite women and their supporters to work together with the supporter holding the woman's hands, maintaining eye contact and asking her to follow his lead in breathing in through the nose and blowing out gently into each other's faces.

TEACHING POSITIONS FOR LABOUR

It is well established in the literature that women who are allowed to move around freely during labour in order to maximize their comfort and who give birth in the position of their choice require less analgesia and have shorter labours than women who are confined to bed and who push their babies out whilst lying flat on their backs or semi-recumbent:

> The results of controlled trial show that women who were asked to stand, walk, or sit upright during labour had, on average, shorter labours than women asked to remain lying flat ... Women allocated to an upright posture used less narcotic analgesics or epidural anaesthesia, and received fewer oxytocics to augment labour.

> Women seem to prefer freedom of movement when it is allowed. Given the opportunity to assume any position in or out of bed during the course of their labour without interference or instruction by care-givers, labouring women spontaneously adopt upright postures such as sitting, standing, and walking. (Enkin et al, 1995, pp 205, 248)

However, the bed still remains the focal point of most delivery rooms, suggesting to women that they should labour and give birth on it. Childbirth educators have a considerable amount of work to do to replace the medical model of birth in which the mother is passive and her carers manage her labour, with a new and dynamic model in which the mother is active and in control of her labour.

The basis of effective teaching about mobility in labour is to ensure that women and their supporters have an elementary understanding of:

- how the pressure of the baby's head on the cervix causes the release of labour hormones

- how the womb rears forwards when it contracts and how much more easily it can do this if the woman is herself upright and leaning forwards

- how the space for the baby in the pelvis is far greater when the woman is standing or kneeling or walking around

Childbirth educators often feel that class attenders are reluctant to leave their seats to try out positions or other practical skills for labour. It is a much easier task to encourage them to undertake some practical work once people are standing. If the educator herself stands up and then invites class members to stand:

(educator stands and says . . .)
'Right – can I ask you all to stand up now please.'

Few, if any, people will refuse. The educator can then move on to her practical skills session:

'In the light of what we've been saying about making as much room as possible for the baby in the pelvis and helping the cervix to open up quickly and evenly, what positions do you think might be useful in labour?'

When a suggestion is made, the educator can invite everyone to try that position and then ask for more suggestions or demonstrate some herself.

While class members are trying out positions for labour, the educator can use a variety of open-ended questions to maintain the momentum and reinforce the relevance of the session:

'How would you feel about being in this position in a hospital delivery room?'

'How do you think your midwife would react if you were in this position?'

'What would it be nice to have in the delivery room to make using different positions easier?'

'What position would you use if you were very tired and had been in labour for a long time?'

'Can you suggest a position that might help with backache?'

'How do you think your baby feels during labour?'

It is easy for labour supporters to feel somewhat at a loose end whilst the women are practising different positions and it is important for the educator to involve them as fully as possible, seeking their opinions and inviting them to imagine what they might be doing during labour:

'What could you do to make the woman more comfortable?'

'Where could you stand or sit in order to have eye contact with the woman or hold her hand if she was in this position?'

'How do you feel about the woman using these positions?'

TEACHING MASSAGE FOR LABOUR

Supporters will doubtless have heard that one of their tasks during labour is to rub the woman's back, and, because this gives them something to do, they are often keen to practise. It is useful for the childbirth educator to introduce massage by enquiring whether anyone in the group has ever had a massage and whether they enjoyed it. Drawing on whatever experience the group has had, the educator can encourage class members to consider how massage should be delivered and what its effects might be during labour. The aim in teaching about massage is to empower supporters to be physically close to the woman in labour even if she is giving birth in an environment which the supporter finds hostile to the expression of intimacy and affection. This empowerment will be effective only if the antenatal class provides the opportunity for supporters to practise holding and touching the woman in ways that will help her relax.

It may feel safer for both the educator and the group to start with a simple massage of a sexually 'neutral' part of the body such as the hand. The educator can ask for a volunteer and demonstrate, perhaps using a base oil such as sweet almond, how to stroke the hand rhythmically, gently pull each finger, massage in small circles over the palm and gently stretch the skin on the back of the hand. The points to make are:

- that the person giving the massage must himself be relaxed if the massage is to be effective

- that during the massage, he must always have physical contact with the person being massaged

- that massage should be smooth and continuous

- that it is important to ask the person being massaged for feedback to ensure that the massage is being provided in the right place and at the right pressure

- that oils are nice for massage, but not essential, and that aromatherapy oils should be used only after consulting with a qualified aromatherapist

- that massage should be enjoyable and, if it is not, it is best either to stop or to try a different kind

If there is sufficient time in the class, it is a good idea for all the group members to have the chance both to give and to receive a massage. As the group's confidence increases, the educator can demonstrate and ask people to practise massage of the shoulders, back, sacrum, hips and thighs, always providing clear explanations of the benefits of massaging these areas during labour (See Fig. 7.3A–E):

Shoulders	if the mother's shoulders are relaxed, she will not over-breathe (hyperventilate)
Back	back massage is especially relaxing in early first stage to help keep calm and conserve energy
Sacrum	contractions are often felt very strongly in the mother's lower back, and providing counter-pressure in this area can help ease the pain
Hips	women sometimes say that they feel their hips are 'coming apart' during labour and it is very comforting to have the hips massaged
Thighs	women may find that their legs become very cold or that their thighs start to wobble in strong labour; stroking firmly down the thighs helps warm them and control the shakiness

PRACTICE CONTRACTIONS

Over the years, childbirth educators have experimented with different ways of simulating contractions in a well meant, but sometimes highly unsuitable, effort to inject realism into their classes. Educators have been known to give women ice-cubes to hold tightly in order to provide a painful stimulus while they practise breathing techniques. Some women have experienced nerve injury as a result. Labour supporters have been asked to give their partners a 'Chinese burn' to mimic the pain of a contraction, or to press down hard on the woman's knees while she is sitting in the tailor position. Such methods are clearly dangerous both physically and perhaps psychologically in that they set up a model of labour supporters (often men) inflicting pain on women.

There are, however, ways of creating physical stress that are safe and can have a dramatic impact on people's understanding of their own coping resources. Stress positions are useful to help class members explore how rhythmical breathing, massage and encouragement can make a physically stressful experience more bearable. One such is the rider position which involves class members standing with their backs against a wall and then sliding down until their thighs are parallel with the floor. (See Fig. 7.4A, B) Over a period of a minute, the ache in the thighs gradually becomes more intense in a way that is not dissimilar to the sensation of a contraction. (See Box 7.8)

It is important to give women and their supporters the opportunity to practise putting together the various skills they have learned for labour whilst imagining contractions. The educator can give people an idea of how long a contraction is, how short the time between contractions may be, and of how contractions build to a peak and then decline using music or

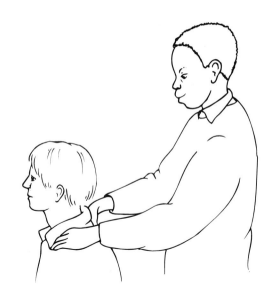

A

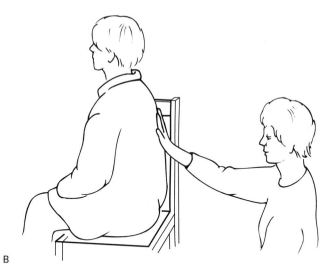

B

FIG. 7.3 A–E.   *(A) Massaging the shoulders. (B) Massaging the back.*

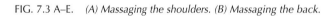

ANTENATAL EDUCATION: A DYNAMIC APPROACH

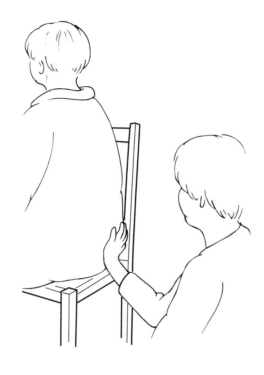

C

D

FIG. 7.3 (Cont'd). *(C) Massaging the sacrum. (D) Massaging the hips.*

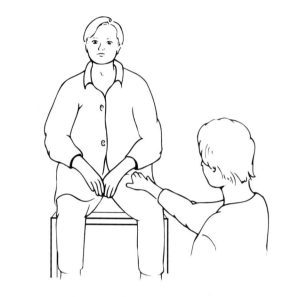

E

FIG. 7.3 (Cont'd).   *(E) Massaging the thighs.*

clapping, which is gradually amplified and then decreased, or by talking people through contractions. In order to become confident to provide such a learning opportunity, the educator needs to practise on her own and with colleagues, conveying the gradually increasing stress of a contraction through the tone of her voice and describing the emotions and sensations that may be felt during a contraction. (See Box 7.9)

It is likely that this exercise, at least on the first occasion when it is practised, will cause a fair amount of giggling and talking. If it also provokes comments such as:

'I'm exhausted already!'

'Not another one!'

'Do they really come as quickly as this?'

'I won't be able to go on rubbing her back for hours!'

then the educator knows that she has provided a good learning experience.

LABOUR REHEARSALS

In the interests of preparing people for labour in as 'real' a manner as possible, the childbirth educator can try to give her group an idea of the possible sequence of events from the onset of labour to the birth of the baby. Describing various labour scenarios and inviting class members to discuss their possible emotions, to think about the decisions they might need to make, and to practise the appropriate skills will facilitate the consolidation of learning achieved during the antenatal course. Labour rehearsals demand that the educator has imagination and a sense of drama, but, if she is sufficiently confident, they provide class members with an excellent learning opportunity. (See Box 7.10)

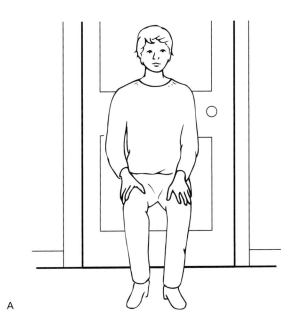

A

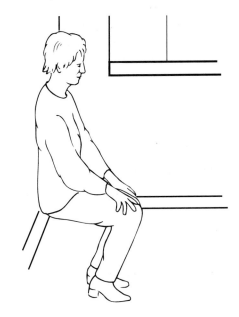

B

FIG. 7.4   *(A, B) Rider position.*

BOX 7.8 COPING WITH STRESS

Aim

* to increase class members' confidence in the efficacy of natural pain control techniques

Learning outcome

* class members will be able to use breathing techniques, massage and verbal encouragement to make physical stress more tolerable

Invite *everyone* to take up the rider position and hold the position for a minute, but emphasize that it is fine to stop before the minute is up if the stress is too great.

Ask for feedback. What happened to people's breathing? What were they thinking about during the exercise?

Now ask people to work in pairs; explain that one person adopts the rider position and the other tries to help her through the minute by massaging her thighs firmly, maintaining eye contact, reminding her to breath rhythmically and offering verbal encouragement.

Time another minute, providing regular updates on how many seconds have passed.

Ask for feedback on whether the position was easier to hold this time and what helped. Comments are likely to include:

* having someone talking to me helped to make the time seem shorter

* rubbing my legs eased the discomfort

* being told how many seconds I had already got through was helpful

* focusing on my breathing helped to distract me

The educator can then draw out the points she wants to make: the importance of support in labour, the usefulness of massage and very simple breathing patterns, and the need to focus on one contraction at a time and to relax during the break in between.

CONCLUSION

Teaching about breathing, massage, relaxation and positions for labour is an exciting part of childbirth preparation classes. The ease with which class members acquire these skills and the likelihood of their being able to use them during labour depend substantially on the educator's confidence to facilitate practical skills work and on her conviction that such skills are effective. Whilst the business of simulating contractions in antenatal classes may seem a million miles from the real experience of the delivery room, it is nevertheless essential that childbirth preparation does not centre exclusively on discussion and information sharing. If it does, the

Box 7.9 Practice Contractions

Aim

• to increase class members' confidence to cope with contractions

Learning outcome

• class members will be able to combine a variety of skills for coping with contractions

Invite the women to take up any position they consider they might use if they were having very strong contractions. Ask supporters to help them get comfortable.

Talk the class through a 'contraction' that lasts 60–90 seconds (timing carefully):

The women can feel a contraction starting now. Take a deep breath, sigh it out and drop your shoulders. The contraction is building up and building up; it's a very strong one – frightening. Focus on relaxing as you breathe out. Drop your shoulders. Supporters are probably anxious that the woman is in a lot of pain and wondering whether everything is going as it should. Just keep massaging her back firmly or talking gently to her. Stay close to her. The women can feel that the contraction is almost at its peak now; it is very strong, the strongest yet. Focus on your out-breath – remember you're breathing for your baby who is also having to cope with this contraction. You might find that you're blowing your breath out quite noisily now, that you want to make a lot of noise. That's all right, but keep the rhythm of your breathing. Focus on the out-breath; drop your shoulders. Supporters – just by being there, you're really helping her to get through this contraction. And it's beginning to ease off now. It's nearly gone now, nearly finished. It's over. (90 seconds)

Now the contraction's finished and all three of you (don't forget your baby) need to relax. Make yourself comfortable. Check that your forehead is smooth, that your jaw is relaxed. Check that your shoulders are loose and low. Make sure that your hands are soft and the fingers curved, not made into a fist.

Does either of you want something to drink or a cool sponge to wipe your face? Look after yourselves.

Relax – don't worry about the contractions. Welcome this break and make the most of it so that you and your baby are ready to cope with the next one. (3 minutes)

There's another contraction starting now. Find a comfortable position. Take a deep breath and relax as you breath out . . .

Box 7.10 Labour Rehearsal

Aims

- to consolidate group members' learning about labour
- to boost parents' confidence to cope with labour

Learning outcomes

Class members will:

- be able to combine skills for coping with labour
- have identified the range of emotions that people have during labour
- have further developed skills of obtaining information and making decisions

Explain that this is a labour rehearsal which will be a mixture of practical work and discussion. Invite class members to participate.

(The following sequence would need to be modified if some members of the group were planning a home birth.)

Describe a possible onset of labour scenario – mother at home with contractions coming at 15-minute intervals; labour supporter elsewhere.

(to the mothers)
How do you feel?

Describe an early first stage contraction while pregnant class members lean on tables or the backs of chairs.

The mother contacts her labour supporter.

(to the labour supporters)
How do you feel when the news arrives that the woman is in labour?

The supporter returns to be with the mother.

How long do you both want to wait before going to the hospital?

Describe a 40-second contraction during the journey to hospital. Invite the women to massage lightly underneath their 'bumps'.

(to the supporters)
How do you feel during this journey?

Mother and supporter arrive at the hospital. After routine admission procedures, they are left alone. Contractions become gradually stronger. The midwife returns and examines the mother who is 6 centimetres dilated. She offers to break the mother's waters.

What information do you need?
What decision will you make?

Describe a strong first stage contraction, lasting 90 seconds. Invite the women to use appropriate positions, to rock their hips, to breathe in through their noses and blow out gently through their mouths. Invite supporters to offer massage, encouragement and reassurance.

(to the supporters)
What could you do to help the woman between contractions?

The mother and her supporter have been in hospital for 5 hours now.

How do you both feel?
Do you want some pain relief?

Second stage has now begun.

Describe a second stage contraction. Invite the women to choose a position that will help their babies to be born easily.

educator runs the risk of suggesting to parents that labour is experienced in the head rather than in the pelvis.

KEY POINTS

1. For psychological, social and political reasons, the aim of antenatal education must be to empower women to trust in their bodies and in their natural ability to give birth to their babies.

2. Antenatal education has a responsibility to enable women to choose a non-medicated delivery as well as informing them about the types of medical pain relief available to them.

3. Many women coming to antenatal classes cannot make a choice about the kind of pain relief they would prefer in labour because they are ignorant of their own resources for coping with pain and of how these can enable the mechanics of labour to work more smoothly.

4. Women cannot learn to work with their bodies by sitting around in discussion groups.

5. Childbirth educators have a considerable amount of work to do to help clients replace the medical model of birth, in which the mother is passive and her carers manage her labour, with a dynamic model in which the mother is active and in control of her labour.

6. Unless the childbirth educator is convinced that women have resources which, in a favourable environment, can enable them to give birth without medical intervention, she is unlikely to convince class members that learning about the resources will be of service to them.

References

Caldeyro-Barcia R (1979) The influence of maternal bearing-down efforts during second stage on fetal well-being. *Birth and the Family Journal* **6**(1): 17–20.

Eggers P (1995) Pain is not a four letter word. *International Journal of Childbirth Education* **10**(4): 4–5.

Enkin M, Keirse MJNC, Renfrew M and Neilson J (1995) *A Guide to Effective Care in Pregnancy and Childbirth*, 2nd edn. Oxford: Oxford University Press.

Nolan M (1996) *Being Pregnant, Giving Birth*. London: HMSO in collaboration with the National Childbirth Trust.

Strychar IM, Griffith WS, Conry RF and Sork TJ (1990) How pregnant women learn about selected health issues: learning transaction types. *Adult Education Quarterly* **41**(1): 17–28.

Thorp JA and Breedlove G (1996) Epidural analgesia in labor: an evaluation of risks and benefits. *Birth* **23**(2): 63–83.

Yerby M (1996) Managing pain in labour. *Modern Midwife* **6**(3): 22–24.

Teaching and Learning About Parenting

8

Childbirth educators may often find themselves teaching courses that include too few hours for there to be sufficient time to cover, either at all or in any great depth, the multiplicity of issues that deserve addressing in relation to the postnatal period. Some who have the luxury of teaching 6- or 8-week courses deliberately choose not to look at postnatal topics in the belief that pregnant parents cannot concentrate on any matters beyond the birth of their babies. Yet to focus antenatal education entirely on the one day in the woman's life when she will be giving birth and to ignore the challenges and complexities of the subsequent 18 years when she, alone or with a partner, will be responsible for preparing a new citizen to take his or her place in society seems bizarre. Government and media repeatedly call for better parenting as a means of tackling the problems in our schools and improving the social behaviour and psychological and sexual health of adolescents, yet there is no strategy for educating people in the skills required to be 'good enough' parents.

For many adults, antenatal classes provide the only opportunity to receive education to prepare them for the immense task of parenting. It is surely not helpful, or ethical, to suggest that the parents' task is accomplished once their baby has been born. Their task is only just beginning. This is not to deny that it is critically important to get birth right for women and their families because women's self-esteem and self-confidence are intimately bound up with their experience of childbirth and their perceptions of how they coped mentally and physically during it (Green et al, 1988; Thune-Larsen and Moller-Pedersen, 1988; Simkin, 1991, 1992). However, birth is the springboard into parenting, and antenatal classes must demonstrate how the skills that people are learning in preparation for labour and birth are also relevant to the first days and weeks of parenting.

It is a myth that parents who are pregnant for the first time cannot project beyond the birth. The agendas that parents set for their classes always include requests for discussion of postnatal topics and for practising babycare skills. Research has found (Hillan, 1992; O'Meara, 1993) that parents criticize their antenatal education when it fails to prepare them for parenting as well as for birth:

Antenatal classes should try and give more of a sense of the experience of having a newborn baby. (Rogers et al, 1996, p 53)

It may be that childbirth educators have used the supposed difficulties of antenatal class attenders in thinking about postnatal life as an excuse for not tackling this huge area. One way of learning about the issues that it might be helpful to look at in classes is to listen to new parents talking about the first months of their babies' lives:

I needed more information about immediately after the birth – coping with the baby in hospital, how to cope at home. Classes should include discussion about your feelings following birth.

I would have liked more insight into emotions and feelings in the first few weeks after birth, also the problems that may be encountered with breastfeeding and that there is no need to feel guilty if you can't cope. It would have been helpful if it was explained how soon things would get back to normal with my husband, especially in relation to touching and breastfeeding. Husbands need to be told what to expect emotionally in the first few weeks from their wives.

Antenatal classes should include practical caring for newborn babies. Realistic talk on how it feels to be parents at first. Postnatal depression.

(interviews recorded by the author, 1995)

Some antenatal groups will include people who have special concerns about the postnatal period. For parents who are disabled, safety issues may be of particular importance; for parents with strong cultural and religious convictions, it may be vital to discuss how traditional and contemporary understanding of babycare and the mother's postnatal recovery can be reconciled; for parents expecting twins or supertwins, the most important issue is how to get the help they will almost certainly need.

Leaving aside these special circumstances (further consideration is given to them in Chapter 10), all prospective parents have concerns in common and these should form the core of antenatal education about the postnatal period. (See Box 8.1)

BOX 8.1 POSTNATAL ISSUES: WHAT DO CLASS ATTENDERS WANT TO KNOW?

Aim

- to raise the awareness of class attenders of their own needs and the needs of their babies in the early postnatal period

Learning outcome

- group members will understand the range of hopes and fears that people have in relation to being parents

In small groups, or in the large group, invite group members to brainstorm three things they are looking forward to about the early weeks with their new babies, and three things they are anxious about.

In the author's experience, the following are the postnatal concerns that are commonly raised in response to this exercise:

- coping with sleepless nights

- understanding why our baby is crying

- having time for myself/ourselves

- division of responsibilities between partners

- financial implications of a new baby

- changes in relationships

- returning to work

- sex after childbirth

- mother's physical and mental health postnatally

It is important when discussing group members' concerns to strike a balance between alerting them to the challenges which life with a new baby involves and fostering their healthy feelings of excitement and happiness about the imminent birth. The childbirth educator, therefore, needs to give due weight to the positive things that people have identified about the early weeks of parenting. These may include:

- becoming a family

- seeing our baby growing and changing

- bathing the baby

- dressing the baby

- feeling I am a proper mother/father now

- not having to wear maternity clothes any more

- watching my partner with the baby

'REAL' BABIES AND 'REAL' PARENTS

One of the factors that prevents pregnant parents from preparing adequately for the postnatal period is the influence of media hype about babies. Childbirth educators face a considerable challenge in enabling parents to replace this powerful mythology with a better understanding of the realities of postnatal life. Realism in antenatal classes does not mean suggesting to parents that there is no joy in the early postnatal period; however, that period is more likely to be joyous if parents have prepared themselves for commonly experienced difficulties and are confident that they have the resources to cope.

An excellent learning opportunity can be created for group members by inviting them to compare the media image of newborn babies with what, from first- or second-hand experience, they know to be the reality. The childbirth educator can use the ensuing discussion to raise issues around postnatal mental health, support and good-enough parenting. (See Box 8.2)

Antenatal classes provide an opportunity for parents to consider what their own needs might be after the birth of their baby, and to plan ahead for how their needs can be met.

BOX 8.2 PERFECT BABIES AND PERFECT PARENTS

Aim

- to protect parents from the stresses caused by unrealistic expectations of babies and parenting

Learning outcome

- group members will have identified facets of normal newborn behaviour and a range of parenting skills

Working in small single-sex or mixed groups, invite group members to write an advert for 'the perfect baby' and 'the perfect parent', followed by brief paragraphs starting: 'Real babies are . . .' and 'Real parents are . . .'

After comparing adverts, the educator can initiate discussion along the lines of:

- Which aspects of the perfect baby would you most like to believe are true?

- Which aspects of the real baby are the most worrying for you?

- What characteristics of the perfect parent would you most like to have?

- What support do you think parents need to make them 'good enough'?

Whereas 100 years ago, when maternal mortality was very high, society's concern was primarily for the well-being of the mother, today the pendulum has swung so far the other way that parents might be excused for thinking that no-one is any longer interested in them, but only in their children. Parents can be compared to jugs of water, expected to pour out their physical and emotional resources into the cups that are their children. There comes a point, however, when the jugs run dry and need replenishing. A group facilitated by the author suggested the following 'needs' of mothers and fathers postnatally:

- time as a couple

- patience

- 'own space'

- sleep

- an escape

- basic knowledge about babycare

- confidence

- time to adjust

- recognition

- to be organized

- flexibility

- financial security

- help with chores

- sense of humour

- baby equipment

- *good* advice

Such a list provides almost endless opportunities for discussion in classes, enabling parents to become assertive in stating their own needs and in identifying and asking for the kind of support they need from health professionals, friends and relatives.

Pregnancy is a time when parents-to-be often reflect on their own upbringing and start to define their ideas about parenting in relation to the way in which they were themselves parented:

> *Psychodynamic theorists would argue that the possible parental self is grounded in one's early years, when identification with one's own parents occurs. Thus, the parenting a person receives as a child ... influences the way he or she parents.* (Antonucci and Mikus, 1988, p 70)

Heightened awareness of the responsibilities that a child brings leads to a re-evaluation by prospective parents of the perceived inadequacies and strengths of their own parents. Encouraging such reflection is one way in which the childbirth educator can help parents move towards defining what will be their own unique parenting style and thereby to achieve greater consistency in parenting than is possible when events in the lives of their babies and children are responded to entirely on an ad hoc basis.

Ice-breakers or small group work can usefully focus on what class attenders consider was particularly good about the way in which they were brought up and how they believe their upbringing could have been improved. From this point, the educator can initiate discussion about what is most important to a child in his/her relationship with parents, why inconsistencies occur in parenting practice and what kind of support parents need to do their job well.

TALKING TO EACH OTHER

Relate counsellors identify failure to talk to each other about the really important issues in their lives as the most common cause of difficulties between partners (Litvinoff, 1991). This may be a result of the pressures and pace of daily living, or of a fear of broaching topics that are likely to cause disagreement. The relationship between a couple survives on a superficial level until a crisis occurs, such as the arrival of a new baby:

> *Parenthood has been found to correlate with increased strain in both men and women ... Early parenthood, in particular, appears to be a time of satisfaction coupled with stress and worry.* (Antonucci and Mikus, 1988, p 64)

At this point, the couple's failure to talk to each other results in each being unable to ask the other for the help and support they require.

Antenatal classes provide a wonderful opportunity for partners to discuss issues that are likely to prove flashpoints later in their parenting careers. The childbirth educator's understanding of small group work needs to embrace the smallest group of all, which is the couple who are coming to classes together. Each class can include a chance for couples to talk to each other on a specific issue that has been highlighted during the class as particularly important. Exercises that enable people to work first on their own and then with their partners are especially useful. (See Boxes 8.3 and 8.4)

BOX 8.3 EXPECTATIONS 1

Aim

- to increase partners' ability to communicate with and to understand each other

Learning outcome

- partners will be able to divide babycare tasks and household chores in a way that both find equitable

Hand everyone in the group the worksheet below and invite people to complete it on their own. After a few minutes, ask partners to compare their lists and discuss any areas of disagreement.

SHARING TASKS

Put ticks in the columns according to whether you think you or your partner will be carrying out the following activities after your baby is born. You may decide that both of you will be doing some things. If this is the case, tick both columns.

	SELF	PARTNER
Feeding the baby	☐	☐
Changing wet nappies	☐	☐
Changing dirty nappies	☐	☐
Bathing the baby	☐	☐
Shopping	☐	☐
Cooking the evening meal	☐	☐
Washing up	☐	☐
Getting up to the baby during the night	☐	☐
Hoovering	☐	☐
Ironing	☐	☐
Carrying the baby in a sling	☐	☐
Pushing the pram	☐	☐
Settling the baby when s/he is crying	☐	☐
Tidying the house	☐	☐

Box 8.4 Expectations 2

Aim

- to increase partners' ability to communicate with and to understand each other

Learning outcome

- partners will know some of the parenting issues that may cause disagreement between them

Circle the number which shows how you feel about the following important parenting issues:

Our baby will share our bed						Our baby will never sleep in our bed			
1	2	3	4	5	6	7	8	9	10

We will never leave our baby to cry						We think it is good for babies to cry for short periods			
1	2	3	4	5	6	7	8	9	10

We will never smack our child						We will smack our child whenever s/he is naughty			
1	2	3	4	5	6	7	8	9	10

We will never allow our child to watch TV						We will allow our child to watch TV every day			
1	2	3	4	5	6	7	8	9	10

Our baby will never eat commercial baby foods						We will use commercial baby foods all the time			
1	2	3	4	5	6	7	8	9	10

We will never be seen naked by our child						We are completely happy for our child to see us naked			
1	2	3	4	5	6	7	8	9	10

We will tell everyone that our child is not allowed to eat sweets						We will never prevent our child from eating sweets			
1	2	3	4	5	6	7	8	9	10

Our child will be brought up as a vegetarian						Our child will have meat every day			
1	2	3	4	5	6	7	8	9	10

Another way of giving couples the opportunity to talk is by offering a few minutes at the end of each topic for them to exchange ideas about what has just been discussed. This enables people who have not spoken in the large group to explain their feelings to their partners, and for couples to consider how coping strategies identified by others might fit into their own lifestyles.

TEACHING APPROACHES TO FACILITATE PROBLEM SOLVING

Pregnant parents are quite able to identify the aspects of life with a new baby that are likely to prove the most challenging. They are also well able to devise appropriate coping strategies based on their observations of other parents and on their own experiences of being brought up with or looking after small children. The childbirth educator's aim is to help people understand how much experience and expertise they already have in the area of childcare and to reassure them that, where experience is lacking, they have sufficient common sense and knowledge of themselves to be able to solve their own problems. It is important for the educator to remember that her job is not to solve parents' difficulties for them, but:

> To give help, support and advice to the extent that the individual mother/family needs and wishes;

> To trust in the parents' will and ability to understand their baby's signals and needs.
> (Kvist et al, 1996, p 87)

Small group work is often a safe way for parents to look at the issues that worry them about the postnatal period and to begin to map out some strategies for coping. Asking people to work together in small groups, rather than in the whole group with the childbirth educator, makes the point that parents can find their own solutions to the inevitable difficulties that are part of life with a new baby and do not have to rely on professional expertise. People can be helped to structure their discussion and explore their ideas in depth if the educator provides some prompts. (See example of worksheet in Box 8.5)

Parents attending one of the author's antenatal courses revealed that they were anxious about how they would cope if their baby cried a lot. They worked in small groups to discuss how they could manage this situation. Their ideas were practical and comprehensive. (See Box 8.6)

Another useful prompt for small group work is the 'situation card' which describes the typical thoughts, feelings and activities of daily living of families with a new baby. Situation cards can be written by the childbirth educator herself to incorporate the concerns she has identified as important to the people in her group. Or, they might consist of the words of new parents themselves. Or they might be quotations taken from books, poems, articles or newspapers. Situation cards can also be used to introduce topics that are often not easy to talk about in classes, such as resuming sexual relations after childbirth, postnatal depression and baby battering. (See Boxes 8.7 and 8.8)

OPPORTUNITIES FOR LEARNING ABOUT CHANGING RELATIONSHIPS

There are a variety of teaching strategies that can be employed to help class members learn from each other about handling relationships so as to minimize conflict and maximize support. Situation cards are useful. The Button Game enables couples to work together to imagine how their social network might be affected by the birth of their baby. (See Box 8.9)

Box 8.5 Sleeping: Parents and Babies

Where is your baby going to sleep at night?

How much unbroken sleep do you expect to get in any 24-hour period during the first weeks of your baby's life?

How will this make you feel?

What effect might this have on

- **your relationship with your partner?**

- **your relationship with your baby?**

Ways of coping with broken nights:

BOX 8.6 IF OUR BABY CRIES A LOT, WE WILL NEED TO:

- Stay calm

- Have a break (put the baby in his/her cot, shut the door and retreat to a place where we cannot hear him/her for a while)

- Try all the different ways we know of soothing him/her (put the baby in a pram and go for a walk; go for a drive; swaddle the baby; play some music; put the baby near the washing machine; massage the baby; bath the baby . . .)

- Ask our midwife/doctor if there's anything wrong with the baby

- Ask other parents for advice

- Hand the baby over to someone else and have a rest/something to eat/go for a walk/have a cry

- Take it in turns with each other or someone else to try to soothe the baby

Last resorts

- Contact CRY-SIS (a support organization which helps parents whose babies cry a lot)

- Consult a cranial osteopath (very good at helping babies who have had difficult births)

BOX 8.7 SITUATION CARDS

Aim

- to promote realistic expectations of the postnatal period

Learning outcome

- group members will know how varied are the feelings and experiences of parents during the early weeks of parenting

Invite people to form small groups and hand each group one or two situation cards. Move round the groups while people are talking, listening (but not contributing) to what is being said in order to find out what topics need further discussion during the course.

BOX 8.8 SITUATION CARDS – EXAMPLES OF SITUATIONS

Health Visitor talking about her baby's sleeplessness:

This sort of thing happened to 'clients' not professionals – didn't it? I turned to family, friends, childcare books – anywhere – for help. The euphoric glow of motherhood faded as I was told I was overfeeding her, underfeeding her, not winding her enough and trying to wind her too hard. Dutifully, I fed her less, fed her more, patted her back, didn't pat her back. We both finished each day utterly exhausted and confused ...

(Jackson, 1990, p 40)

Sheer exhaustion can often delay the return of sexual relations. After a day filled with dirty nappies, feeding a crying baby, unwanted visitors, perineal pain and no peace and quiet, the last thing a new mother would have in mind is energetic love-making, however much she may love her partner. The only cure for tiredness is sleep, which should be taken when the baby chooses to sleep. Having intercourse when both parties are awake and interested may be the simple solution, as often bedtime does not coincide with this.

(Evans, 1992, p 17)

I love being a mother to this tiny little baby. I love being a parent. Geoff hates it. He finds it really difficult. He wakes up in the morning sometimes and the baby's crying and he groans and says, 'Oh no'. He wishes the baby was ... well, if not there, not born yet. Or that there was someone else to look after him. He feels the baby gets between us and interferes.

(McGrail, 1996, p 135)

I found myself having negative feelings towards the child when he was born. It was only in retrospect that you recognise this, and how a good birth helps you, even a man, bond more readily than when you get a really awful institutional birth. It can have a bad effect on you. It doesn't help you start off very well.

(Rogers et al, 1996, p 51)

> *Susan was a particularly house-proud mother. Her house was beautifully kept and by dint of enormous hard work she maintained high standards despite her young twins ... the babies were always dressed immaculately and neatly kept in bouncer chairs or a playpen. Not a thing was out of place, not even the twins.*
>
> *By the time the babies reached their first birthday, Susan sadly realised she had spent so much time on housework that she had not allowed herself to enjoy the babies – nor they her. She saw that precious cuddling time could never be recovered.*
>
> (Bryan, 1984, p 83)

BOX 8.9 CHANGING RELATIONSHIPS

Aim:

* to increase parents' ability to manage relationships after the birth of their babies

Learning outcome

* parents will have identified the part played by important people in their lives now and the part they may play after the birth of their babies

Make available a pile of buttons of different shapes and colours. Invite each woman and her supporter to take a handful. One button is selected to represent the couple (or mother). The rest represent the important people in their lives and each is placed closer to the 'couple button' or farther away depending on the importance of that person to them.

When the current pattern of relationships has been laid out in this way, another button is chosen to represent the baby. Couples then consider how the 'baby button' will alter the position of other buttons in the pattern.

Role play can be an excellent way of exploring how relationships may change after the birth of a new baby, although it needs to be made 'safe' for class attenders, most of whom will be resistant to any idea that they should participate in acting. Techniques of role play which involve people having to say very little are usually the most successful; sometimes what starts as a silent role play develops into an extended dialogue as participants become more confident in their roles. (See Box 8.10)

A role play such as 'Family Photographs' can elicit strong feelings and requires the childbirth educator to be very aware of how people are responding to the roles they have assumed and whether anyone is becoming distressed. From a position of empathy with the significant others in their social and familial group, parents can discuss what they can

Box 8.10 Family Photographs
(Relationships before and after the birth of a baby)

Aim

- to increase parents' ability to manage relationships after the birth of their babies

Learning outcome

- group members will understand ways in which their baby will influence their relationship with other people

After splitting into small groups of six or eight, invite class attenders to choose one of the following roles. One person needs to be the 'new mother'.

'new' mother; 'new' father; maternal grandmother; maternal grandfather; paternal grandmother; paternal grandfather; mother's best friend; mother's employer; father's best friend; father's employer; and any other people whom the group consider significant in their lives.

Invite group members to complete the following sentences from the point of view of their chosen role. Ask them to write down their immediate responses without thinking too closely and without conferring with each other.

I am (the person whose role I am playing)

Now that the baby is born, I feel . . . .

I would like . . . .

I would not like . . . .

Sometimes, it seems . . . .

The baby is . . . .

When everyone has completed their sentences, ask group members to decide the order they are going to speak in, and then to stand together as if for a photograph with each person considering where he or she should be in relation to the new mother.

Ask people to read out, in the order they have already agreed, the first sentence they have completed. Then each person reads out his or her second sentence, third sentence and so on.

Discuss the way in which everyone within the parents' social network is affected more or less immediately by the arrival of their baby. Invite group members to share any insights they have gained from the exercise.

reasonably expect from each other after the birth of their baby and what other people might reasonably expect of them. Anticipating possible difficulties in postnatal relationships enables parents to think ahead so as to be able to diffuse tensions that may arise.

SUPPORT AND MENTAL HEALTH

The importance of social support following childbirth cannot be underestimated:

> *Those mothers who were relatively unsupported in the early stages of motherhood were more likely to become depressed than those with a more supportive social network.* (McIntosh, 1993, p 248)

Childbirth educators need to help clients examine their social networks and identify where their support will come from after the arrival of their babies (Polomeno, 1996). Some women who are giving up full-time jobs in order to care for their babies may find themselves cut off from friendships that were dependent on their involvement in the workplace. Some women or couples live far away from their families. Others may recently have moved house and district. Others again may be isolated as a result of disability, ethnicity or youth. Some people with whom expectant couples are currently in a close relationship will distance themselves once the couples' availability for socializing is reduced as a result of childcare responsibilities. Others, however, will be delighted to play a more significant role in the life of the new family (Gottlieb and Pancer, 1988).

Research suggests that what parents most urgently require in the first weeks of their babies' lives is practical assistance with babycare tasks, household work, shopping and food preparation (Gottlieb and Pancer, 1988). Visitors who expect to be waited on and wish only to cuddle the baby without contributing anything to the management of the household are a source of irritation and distress. Conflicting advice is extremely unwelcome as it threatens the confidence of the mother and father at a time when they are only just starting to understand their baby's signals and are extremely vulnerable to suggestions that they may not be providing the best care for their baby.

Because the incidence of postnatal depression is currently so high – longitudinal studies suggest that 8–14% of women have a depressive neurosis at 3 months' postpartum (Cox, 1986) – and because vulnerability factors can be anticipated in the antenatal period, it is vital for childbirth educators to include postnatal mental health on their class agendas. Until quite recently, the favoured model of postnatal depression was one that stressed biological and psychological factors as causative agents. This model has been challenged by research into social factors influencing depression and it is now thought that the absence of support networks, poor marital relationships, low levels of knowledge about childcare and major life events of the kind that often accompany childbirth (change in financial status, stopping work, revision of personal habits, sexual difficulties) are highly significant in the development of postnatal depression (Kendall et al, 1981; Cooper and Stein, 1989).

Childbirth educators can play a part in helping parents protect themselves against postnatal depression by educating for parenting as well as for birth. The areas that it is vital for parents to consider in advance of the birth of their babies are:

1. Support networks

- how relationships will change after the birth

- help available from health professionals

- contact with other mothers/fathers with small children

- childcare arrangements
- community resources for parents with small children

2. Prioritizing

- household tasks
- sleeping
- eating
- time without the baby

3. Communication with partner

It is important to enable parents to explore their personal support network and to consider ways in which it might be strengthened. The following questionnaire can be completed by each individual on his or her own, and then discussed in partner or non-partner pairs. (See Box 8.11)

Most of the work done by the childbirth educator to help parents remain mentally healthy after their babies are born is embedded in the fabric of her teaching. The way in which she values the contribution made by each person, the respect she accords to every question asked, the way in which she helps group members appreciate how much knowledge and experience they already have to help them through the transition to parenthood – all these build individuals' self-esteem and thereby make them less vulnerable to depression.

Group members also need to learn about postnatal illness and to receive information, if they do not already have it, about the kinds of treatment that are currently available. One of the most important points about postnatal depression for people to understand is that it is a fluid concept and that the symptoms that may characterize one person's depression may not be the same as those experienced by another. Knowing when to seek help depends on recognizing changes in mood and habits. Having a baby brings so many changes into a woman's or a couple's life that the problem is to recognize when the changes that are occurring are in excess of what might be expected following the birth of a baby. (See Box 8.12)

Talking About 'Difficult' Postnatal Topics

Loss and grief in childbirth

There are a number of topics that need to be raised in antenatal classes but which it is difficult to talk about. The difficulty generally lies both with the childbirth educator herself and with the group members. Ours is a society that handles issues around disability and death with considerable reserve; we are ill at ease with disabled people and with those who have suffered a bereavement. The UK infant mortality rate is now so low (6.1 per 1000 live births: Hansard: 18 June 1996, Col 412) that the death of a new baby is not the everyday event it would have been in the lives of our great grandparents. Antenatal screening can test for a wide range of disabilities and is offered in the expectation that parents will choose to abort their fetus if a problem is discovered. Parents who give birth to a disabled baby after making a decision not to abort are often considered odd or even perverted, and those who give birth to a baby whose disability was not detected in utero are pitied. The quest for the perfect baby has proceeded so far that it is becoming increasingly difficult for parents whose baby is disabled or who dies to cope with the gulf between their expectations of birth and the reality with which they are confronted.

BOX 8.11 SUPPORT NETWORKS

After your baby is born, you will probably want to talk to other people about how you are feeling and how your life has changed. Perhaps the person you will talk to most will be your partner. However, your partner may not always be available, or he or she may not be the right person to discuss certain things with, or you may not have a partner. Different needs can be met by different people.

Look at this list and write down the names of people whom you think you could turn to:

	First person	Second person
Someone who accepts me as I am		
Someone reliable in a crisis		
Someone who will tell me honestly what he or she thinks		
Someone who will challenge me when I'm not behaving sensibly		
Someone who is stimulating to be with		
Someone who is good fun to be with		
Someone whom I can trust with very private details about my life		
Someone who makes me feel good about myself		
Someone to talk to when I feel depressed, who will understand and not gossip		

A whole group discussion can be initiated by the educator to look at ways of strengthening support:

- Will these people be available during the day when you are at home with your baby?

- Are they people with children themselves? Will they be interested in how you feel as a parent?

- What support groups are there for parents in your area?

Nobody would deny that parents whose birth outcome is different from the normal one need support. Childbirth educators who enjoy accompanying people through the transition to parenthood must also be prepared to help when the transition is to becoming parents of a disabled baby or of a baby who dies. This means that antenatal classes cannot, as society so often does, sweep the issues of death and disability under the carpet. Classes must model acceptance of such outcomes and a willingness to talk about them and offer support.

BOX 8.12 EXPLORING POSTNATAL DEPRESSION

Aim

- to deepen group members' understanding of postnatal depression

Learning outcomes

- group members will know what are the significant changes associated with postnatal depression

- group members will know some strategies for minimizing their risk of postnatal depression

On a table, place three header cards labelled:

'Normal'   '?'   'Depressed'

Have prepared a pile of small cards, each describing one symptom possibly associated with depression such as:

'avoids other people'; 'unresponsive'; 'hopeless'; 'thoughts of suicide'; 'feels low, especially early in the day'; 'no appetite'; 'losing weight'; 'occasional panic attacks'; 'finds it hard to get to sleep'; 'wakes early and can't get back to sleep'; 'shaky'; 'can't bear baby crying'; 'poor concentration'; 'tearful'; 'can't think clearly'; 'craves sweets and chocolate'; 'always tired'; 'worries about small things'; 'aches and pains'; 'headaches'; 'irritable'; 'feels guilty'; 'feels incompetent'; 'feels worthless'.

Give a few cards to each member of the group. Ask everyone in turn to read out one card and place it under the heading of 'normal', '?' or 'depressed'.

It is likely that there will be much discussion regarding the correct positioning of the cards, with people disagreeing about what can be considered normal following the birth of a baby and what is abnormal. The educator can draw out of the discussion key points such as:

- the symptoms of postnatal depression may be different for different people

- excessive tiredness and social isolation may account for many symptoms of depression and these are the first things to tackle if a new parent is feeling low

- if the mother is depressed, her partner is at risk of depression

- it may be difficult to know whether someone is clinically depressed, but parents should not hesitate to seek help from their Health Visitor or GP if they are feeling low

- antidepressants are not addictive, and combined drug and counselling therapy is generally successful in helping women and couples overcome depression and enjoy a normal, fulfilling life as parents.

It is, however, very difficult to broach the subject of unexpected birth outcomes in a group of happily expectant parents who confront their worst fears about birth only in their dreams. Childbirth educators, especially if they are also the parents of healthy children, often feel guilty about raising issues that may upset and perhaps frighten people. It is important that they should have thoroughly debriefed their own first- or second-hand experiences of stillbirth, cot death and disability before attempting to provide learning opportunities for clients on these topics. Only when the educator understands the sources of her own reluctance, if it exists, to handle such issues is she in a position to help her clients face their fears.

Some childbirth educators like to programme into their course a particular activity to enable people to think about stillbirth and disability; others prefer to wait for an opportunity provided by the group members themselves. Such opportunities nearly always arise. Someone may mention having seen an upsetting programme about sick or disabled children or children dying, or reveal during an exercise about the joys and difficulties of parenting that he or she dreads being the parent of a disabled child. It is generally easier for groups to talk about difficult topics when the seeds of discussion have been sown in such a spontaneous manner.

There are, however, a variety of useful exercises that provide a formal opportunity for parents to think about different birth outcomes. The emphasis during any discussion which ensues as a result of these learning activities needs to be on the kind of support that parents require if their baby is unwell, disabled or dies at birth, and where that support might be available from. (See Box 8.13)

It is very difficult to allow parents *time* to confront the possibility that their baby might be born with a serious disability or be ill at birth or die, and to *wait* for someone to open up a discussion about how they would feel and what they would need in those circumstances. The temptation for the childbirth educator is to break into the inevitable silences and fill them up with words. However, if it is her aim to present as realistic a picture as possible of what it is like to have a baby, the picture she paints must include the darker shades that accurately represent some people's experience of childbearing. Should any of her clients experience an unhappy birth outcome, it is more likely that they will feel able to seek support from both her and from other parents in the group if the possibility of birth tragedies has been openly accepted during classes.

The account of the 'Holiday to Italy' might serve as another approach to the topic of unexpected outcomes. It could be the focus for small group work, or it could be given to couples to look at and discuss with each other, or it could be read out to the whole group by the childbirth educator. (See Box 8.14)

Discussion of loss and grief in childbirth can also embrace how class attenders might feel if the sort of birth they are planning for does not materialize. Some people may be very disappointed if their labour is not completely natural and their baby needs help in the form of ventouse or forceps or caesarean section to be born. It may be extremely upsetting for a woman who really wants to breastfeed her baby to find she has such difficulties that bottle-feeding becomes the only option. The childbirth educator needs to acknowledge the range of childbearing losses that may be experienced and to reassure class attenders that it is no shame to grieve over events that others may see as trivial.

Any discussion about different birth outcomes may precipitate distress on the part of members of the group. Some people may cry or leave the room. It is important for the childbirth educator to accept these reactions as natural and to acknowledge how difficult the topic is. She may need quietly to put an arm round someone who starts crying during the discussion, recognizing, but not trying to control, their sadness. Very often, group members who have become close over a number of weeks will offer each other the support that is needed. People may state that they want to end the discussion or that they feel it is morbid,

---

BOX 8.13 LOSS AND GRIEF IN CHILDBIRTH

Aim

- to heighten awareness of the feelings and needs of parents whose baby is stillborn, not healthy at birth or disabled

Learning outcome

- group members will know what kinds of support are available to parents whose baby is stillborn, not healthy at birth or disabled, and how to access support

On a flipchart, draw a large flower with as many petals as there are people in the antenatal group, and a thick stem.

Invite people to write on the petals the things such as 'patience' or 'sense of humour' that they would like their babies to have. Ask them to write on the stem the things that parents need in order to be able to look after themselves and their children.

Read out what everyone has written and acknowledge the range of attributes identified by the group. Then choose a petal which says 'good health' (there is almost bound to be one), cover it up and ask parents how they would feel if their baby was born without this particular attribute.

Wait as long as is necessary for someone to answer.

Ask what support parents would need if their baby was born without normal health.

Wait as long as is necessary for someone to answer.

Group members will identify that parents would need exactly the same support as the parents of a healthy baby, only to a much greater extent. They are also likely to suggest specific support measures such as contacting the organization for the particular disability the baby has, finding out from specialist health professionals what treatment is required if the baby is poorly, and talking to other parents whose baby has died or has been born unwell or disabled. Write these extra support measures on leaves attached to the stem of the flower (Fig. 8.1).

---

and it is important for the childbirth educator to recognize that a very brief discussion may be sufficient for one group whereas another wants to talk at greater length.

Sex after Childbirth

Discussion about love-making in the early postnatal period will be more useful if group members understand how a woman's body changes and recovers after giving birth. Women are frequently surprised to find out, for example, that vaginal bleeding may continue for weeks, that their breasts may be tender whether they are breastfeeding or not, that stitches

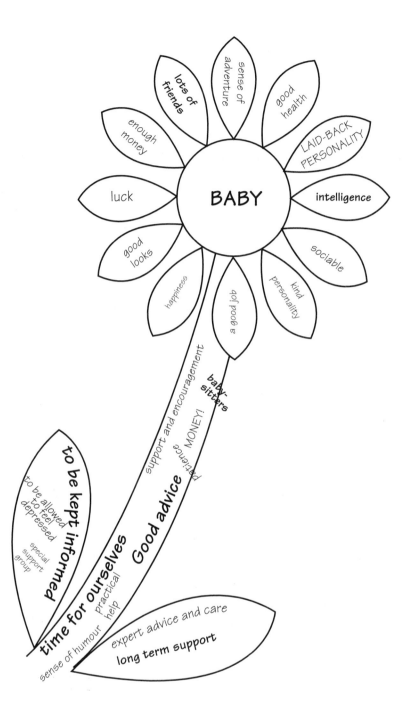

FIG. 8.1 *Flip chart exercise to illustrate support measures needed for parents whose baby is stillborn, not healthy at birth, or disabled.*

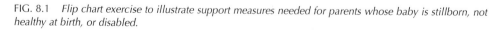

ANTENATAL EDUCATION: A DYNAMIC APPROACH

BOX 8.14 HOLIDAY TO ITALY

(Part of a speech given by Diane Crutcher, Director, to the USA Down's Syndrome Association)

When you are going to have a baby, it is like you are planning a holiday in Italy. You are all excited – you get a lot of guide books and you learn a few phrases in Italian so you can get around. When the time comes, you pack your bags and head for the airport to catch your flight to Italy. Only when you land and the stewardess says 'Welcome to Holland' do you look at one another in disbelief and shock and say 'Holland?' What are you talking about? I booked for Italy.

They then explain that there has been a change of plans and you have landed in Holland where you have to stay. 'But I don't know anything about Holland!' you say. 'I don't want to stay.' But you do – you go out and buy some new guide books. You learn some new phrases and you meet new people. The important thing is that you are not in a filthy, plague-infested slum full of pestilence and famine. You are simply in a different place from the one you had planned. It is slower-paced than Italy and less flashy, but after you have been there a while and you have had a chance to catch your breath, you begin to discover that Holland has windmills, Holland has tulips, Holland has Rembrandts!

Of course, everyone you know is busy coming and going to Italy. They are all bragging about what a great time they had there and for the rest of your life, you will say, 'Yes, that's where I was going. That's what I planned!' The pain of that will never, ever, go away. You have to accept that pain because the loss of that dream, the loss of that plan, is a very, very significant loss. But if you spend your life mourning the fact that you did not get to Italy, you will never be free to enjoy the very special, the very lovely things about Holland.

may take a long time to heal and that regaining their pre-pregnancy weight may not happen within a few months even if they are breastfeeding. These are all areas that can be broached in any discussion focusing on the changes in parents' lives after their babies are born.

Before she can successfully facilitate discussion about sexuality, the childbirth educator needs to have reflected on her own attitudes towards sex and her own experiences of sex after childbirth (Lief and Payne, 1975). While these remain unacknowledged and unexplored, they are likely to colour her approach to this sensitive issue, possibly to the detriment of the learning opportunity she is trying to provide for her group. Some educators, perhaps many, find themselves unable to discuss sexual issues during classes and need to challenge themselves about this:

> *It appears that few midwives routinely discuss the resumption of sexual relations after childbirth with couples – it seems rarely to be talked about in parentcraft education classes and scantily mentioned, if ever, on the postnatal ward.* (Evans, 1992, p 14)

Marital disharmony after childbirth can be precipitated by unsatisfactory sex or the unwillingness of either partner to have sexual relations. Childbirth education programmes which aim to assist parents in making the transition to emotionally fulfilling parenthood need to acknowledge the importance of sexuality in people's lives (Robson et al, 1981).

It is important for childbirth educators to identify from reading the literature, and talking to other educators and to parents, the important aspects of postnatal sexuality that parents need to be aware of. Such a list might include:

- when to resume love-making: after a normal delivery/assisted delivery/caesarean section

- painful intercourse: causes and solutions

- breastfeeding and intercourse

- talking to each other about sexual feelings and needs

- contraception

Parents who are part of a group whose members have got to know each other well, who are accustomed to having their ideas respected by the educator and their questions answered, may well raise sexual issues themselves. At the end of such a discussion, it is helpful to provide partners with a few moments to exchange ideas and feelings with each other.

Situation cards can be used to help people think about sexual matters. (See Box 8.15)

Box 8.15

Jane's and Matt's baby is 8 weeks old. Jane is breastfeeding, which she finds very satisfying. She is fully recovered from the birth and, apart from feeling tired, is fit and well. However, she doesn't want to make love, feeling totally fulfilled by her baby. Matt is ready to start love-making, but senses Jane's reluctance. He wonders how long it will be before he can expect to have a regular sex life again.

Teaching pelvic floor muscle exercises is an ideal opportunity to help couples think about their sexual relationship. Men and women will be interested to learn that one of the best ways for the woman to test her pelvic floor muscles is during intercourse. Postnatal 'goody bags' are also an innovative way of introducing sexual topics into antenatal classes. (See Box 8.16)

'Talking Heads' can be used to help group members think about complex issues such as changes in relationships after the birth of a baby or to broach topics that group members may find it difficult to discuss freely, such as sexuality. (See Box 8.17)

Returning to Work

Although 'returning to work' is included under the heading of 'difficult topics' in this chapter, it is not really difficult to talk about in classes; however it is frequently neglected. Formal antenatal education dates back to a time when women gave up work to become mothers and stayed at home to raise their families to adulthood. This has clearly changed, with a majority of women now returning to the workforce soon after the birth of their babies. Childbirth education has generally failed to acknowledge this change in the pattern of women's lives.

Society still finds itself very much in two minds about women who return to work after giving birth, on the one hand arguing for a woman's right to pursue a career and be financially independent, on the other implying that at least half the problems in children's and young

---

BOX 8.16 POSTNATAL GOODY BAG

Aim

- to prepare group members for the realities of parenting

Learning outcome

- group members will be familiar with some of the practical and emotional issues relating to the postnatal period

Put into a pillow slip a range of items connected with early parenting – terry nappy, disposable nappy, pacifier, baby alarm, cat net, packet of contraceptive pills, tube of KY jelly, condom, breast pads, jar of baby food, scratch mittens, list of films showing at the local cinema, room thermometer, talcum powder etc.

Pass the pillow slip round the group, inviting everyone to take one item and to talk about the ideas it brings to mind.

Items such as contraceptives, breast pads and KY jelly can be used to initiate discussion about sex after childbirth. The group may cover all the important issues themselves or the educator can prompt with questions such as: 'How do you think breastfeeding might affect your love life?' 'What do you think might worry you about starting to have sex again after your baby is born?' 'How long do you think you should wait before making love?'

---

people's lives are caused by mothers going out to work. Women who do choose to stay at home are often not supported in their decision either, losing status when they give up their jobs and encountering criticism that they are failing to achieve their full potential. Antenatal classes can provide an excellent opportunity for parents to explore where they stand in the debate and to identify what support they need, whether returning to work or not.

The following questionnaires might form the basis of small group work. They enable the childbirth educator to raise issues about changes in identity when a woman becomes a mother, managing isolation at home, employment options, family finances and the partner's role. (See Boxes 8.18 and 8.19)

If the majority of women in the class are choosing to return to work after their babies are born, the educator needs to help them identify the important practical issues they need to think about. A typical list might include:

- time management

- balancing the needs of work, partner, baby, self

- childcare arrangements

- expressing and storing breast milk

- changing from breastfeeding to bottle-feeding

- expressing breast milk at work

BOX 8.17 'TALKING HEADS'

Aim

*   to enable parents to communicate their feelings more effectively

Learning outcome

*   group members will know what kinds of emotions men and women may feel in relation to some common postnatal situations

On several large sheets of paper, draw 'heads' (which can be neutral in terms of gender or include features that suggest gender).

At the top of each sheet, write a brief scenario; for example:

It is four weeks since your baby was born. Your partner wants to make love tonight . . .

Your baby is spending her third day in the Special Care Baby Unit; she is needing help to breathe and is being fed by a tube . . .

You have just come home from work and your partner is pacing the kitchen floor with a screaming baby . . .

Give group members marker pens (one colour for the men and another for the women) and ask them to write down inside the 'head' their immediate thoughts in response to each situation.

Then invite people to write down some coping strategies outside the heads.

BOX 8.18 RETURNING TO WORK/STAYING AT HOME

Going back to work

What is the image of the working mother in our society?
What are the advantages if the mother goes back to work after the birth of her baby?
What are the drawbacks?
What can employers do to help women combine work and parenting?
What support do the women in this group need if they go back to work?

Home-making

What is the image of the home-maker mother in our society?
What are the advantages if a mother stays at home to look after her baby?
What are the drawbacks?
What support do the women in this group need if they choose to stay at home?

(adapted from Walter, 1996)

BOX 8.19 FACT OR FICTION?

How do you feel about the following statements?

- Women who have families and careers are 'superwomen' while mothers who stay at home are throwbacks to the 1950s.

- Women who are home-makers spend most of their day on household chores and have a lot of spare time.

- Few women would choose to stay at home to look after their children.

- Home-makers are lonely and their children are short of opportunities to mix with other children.

- Women fall into one of two separate camps – those at home and those in the work force.

- Women have the choice to be home-makers only if they have well-paid partners.

(adapted from Walter, 1996)

CONCLUSION

Antenatal classes provide a golden opportunity for expectant parents to prepare themselves for the adjustments that the arrival of a new baby necessitates. People come to classes anticipating that they will learn about labour and birth; if asked, they are nearly always keen to learn about parenting as well. The skill of the childbirth educator in providing learning opportunities about the postnatal period may play a significant part in improving people's experience of early parenting and, more generally, in improving the quality of parenting in our society.

KEY POINTS

1. Research suggests that parents want antenatal education to prepare them for parenting as well as for birth.

2. Class attenders need to separate the media hype around babies from the realities of parenting young children.

3. Childbirth educators can help parents examine their social networks and identify where their support will come from after the arrival of their babies.

4. Group work in antenatal classes models how parents can find solutions within their own peer group to many of the problems they will encounter postnatally.

TEACHING AND LEARNING ABOUT PARENTING

143

5. Antenatal classes model acceptance of loss and grief in childbirth by including discussion of stillbirth, disability, cot death and less than perfect birth experiences.

References

Antonucci TC and Mikus K. (1988) The power of parenthood: personality and attitudinal changes during the transition to parenthood. In Michaels GY and Goldberg WA (eds) *The Transition to Parenthood: Current Theory and Research*, pp 62–84. Cambridge: Cambridge University Press.

Bryan EM (1984) Twins in the family: a parent's guide. London: Constable.

Cooper PJ and Stein A (1989) Life events and postnatal depression: the Oxford study. In Cox J, Paykel E and Page ML (eds) *Current Approaches: Childbirth as a Life Event*. Dorchester: Duphar Medical Relations.

Cox J (1986) *Postnatal Depression: A Guide for Health Professionals*. London: Churchill Livingstone.

Evans K (1992) Getting back to nature. *Modern Midwife* **January/February**: 14–17.

Gottlieb BH and Pancer SM (1988) Social networks and the transition to parenthood. In Michaels GY and Goldberg WA (eds) *The Transition to Parenthood: Current Theory and Research*, pp 235–269. Cambridge: Cambridge University Press.

Green M, Coupland VA and Kitzinger JV (1988) *Great Expectations: A Prospective Study of Women's Expectations and Experiences of Childbirth*, Vol. 1. Cambridge: University of Cambridge, Child Care and Development Group.

Hillan E (1992) Issues in the delivery of midwifery care. *Journal of Advanced Nursing*, **17**: 274–278.

Jackson D (1990) Three in a bed. London: Bloomsbury.

Kendall RE, Rennie D, Clarke JA and Dean C (1981) The social and obstetric correlates of psychiatric admission in the puerperium. *Psychological Medicine* **11**: 341–360.

Kvist LJ, Persson E and Lingman GK (1996) A comparative study of breast feeding after traditional postnatal hospital care and early discharge. *Midwifery* **12**: 85–92.

Lief H and Payne T (1975) Sexuality – knowledge and attitudes. *American Journal of Nursing* **75**: 2026–2029.

Litvinoff S (1991) *The Relate Guide to Better Relationships*. London: Ebury Press.

McGrail A (1996) Becoming a family. Cambridge: HMSO in collaboration with NCT Publishing.

McIntosh J (1993) The experience of motherhood and the development of depression in the postnatal period. *Journal of Clinical Nursing* **2**: 243–249.

O' Meara C (1993) A diagnostic model for the evaluation of childbirth and parenting education. *Midwifery* **9**: 28–34.

Polomeno V (1996) Social support during pregnancy. *International Journal of Childbirth Education* **11**(2): 14–21.

Robson KM, Brant HA and Kumar R. (1981) Maternal sexuality during first pregnancy and after childbirth. *British Journal of Obstetrics and Gynaecology* **88**: 882–889.

Rogers A, Pilgrim D and Latham M (1996) Understanding and Promoting Mental Health: A Study of Familial Views. London: Health Education Authority.

Simkin P (1991) Just another day in a woman's life? Women's long-term perceptions of their first birth experience. Part 1. *Birth* **18**(4): 203–210.

Simkin P (1992) Just another day in a woman's life? Part II: Nature and consistency of women's long-term memories of their first birth experiences. *Birth* **19**(2): 64–81.

Thune-Larsen K and Moller-Pedersen K (1988) Childbirth experience and postpartum emotional disturbance. *Journal of Reproductive and Infant Psychology* **6**: 229–240.

Walter BE (1996) Childbirth educators can assist new mothers in the stay-at-home choice. *International Journal of Childbirth Education* **11**(1): 31–35.

Learning Opportunities for Men in Antenatal Classes

9

MEN'S ROLE IN LABOUR AND AT THE BIRTH

Organizations such as the Association for Improvements in the Maternity Services and the National Childbirth Trust were campaigning for men to be allowed into the delivery room and had largely achieved this objective several years before antenatal education caught up with the fact that men might welcome some preparation for their new role as labour companions. The presence of men in the delivery rooms of Western hospitals represents a cultural phenomenon that is entirely new. In traditional communities, it is unheard of for men to be present while women give birth (Raphael, 1973). Women expect to be supported during labour by women who are themselves mothers or who have previously assisted at births. The radical shift in the Western philosophy of birth, from seeing it as a family-centred, intimate and everyday event to fearing it as a time in a woman's life when she requires access to the most advanced technology and the closest medical supervision, means that women now give birth in an alien environment, surrounded by people whom they do not know. The woman-to-woman support that the birthing mother once found within her own community is no longer available. It is under these circumstances that women have turned to their male partners to provide the support they need during labour.

Whilst many men (but by no means all) are keen to be present at the birth of their child, it should be remembered that they do not share a gender-based understanding or deep-rooted cultural consciousness of what birth is about and what kind of support the birthing woman might need. Some men, by virtue of either upbringing or personality, are able to enter wholeheartedly into the woman's experience and demonstrate an instinctive understanding of what will help her during labour. Others are ill at ease in the delivery room, unsure about their role, resentful of pressure to accompany their partner when their desire is to be elsewhere:

Men sometimes find it hard to observe, accept, and understand a woman's instinctive behaviour during childbirth. Instead, they often try to keep her from slipping out of a rational, self-controlled state. (Odent, 1994, p 43)

These men are not 'failures'; indeed, they are far more representative of the role men have historically played in childbirth than those who choose to be present at birth and are happy and comfortable to be so.

It is generally accepted that women who are well supported during labour and birth have better physical and emotional outcomes than those who are not. The evidence in support of this contention comes from several famous studies, the first of which was Sosa's and Kennell's Guatemalan study carried out in 1980 (Sosa et al, 1980). The researchers were concerned that women from rural communities coming to the large maternity hospital in Guatemala City to give birth to their babies were experiencing very protracted labours. They recognized that, while the women enjoyed far better standards of medical attention than they would have received in their own communities, they did *not* have the support during labour of another woman experienced in childbirth as they would have done at home. They wondered whether providing the women with this kind of support would affect the length of their labours. To test this hypothesis, they offered one group of primiparous women continuous support during labour from women who were themselves mothers, and another group normal hospital care which included intermittent support from a midwife during first stage and continuous attention during second. The women supporters were called 'doulas', a Greek word describing an older woman who assists a new mother during childbirth and in the first weeks of her baby's life. By this simple intervention, the average length of labour was reduced to 8 hours in the supported group from 19 hours in the control group. Moreover, 26% of control mothers required caesarean sections and 16% augmentation of labour compared with 6% and 2% of the supported group.

The literature has been less conclusive about the effectiveness of men as labour supporters. Bertsch et al (1990) compared the support offered during labour by doulas and fathers, and found that, whereas doulas stroked, rubbed and held the labouring woman more than 95% of the time, fathers did so for less than 20% of the time. Chapman's study (1992) of 20 couples of different racial origin found that the role most commonly adopted by fathers during labour was that of witness rather than coach or team-mate, and concluded that current expectations of the support fathers can offer during childbirth should be re-evaluated.

If it is unreasonable to ask men to provide the intimate, instinctual support that a woman can provide for another woman during labour, it is none the less important to help them understand what support activities they might engage in if they choose to do so and to prepare them for what they will see and hear during labour. The education of men during the antenatal period reflects the gradual shift in maternity care since the 1970s from woman-centred to family-centred care. The woman and her baby are not now seen as an isolated unit, but as defined by and dependent on their relationship with significant others. The most significant of these is likely to be the man who is the baby's father and the woman's partner. Peterson and Walls (1991) summarize the new goal of antenatal education as it strives to meet the needs of men attending classes:

> Paternal–infant bonding should be promoted along with maternal–infant bonding and the goal be fostering strong family bonds ... No individual is more likely to be concerned about the well-being of mother and baby than the father. When considering labor support, there must also be support of the integrity of the family unit. (p 38)

The new family is created when the woman shares the news of her pregnancy with her partner. From this point, the father's experiences of pregnancy and childbirth are likely to be as influential in shaping his relationship with his child as are the mother's in shaping hers (Duncan and Markman, 1988). Whatever role he plays during labour, the father's participation in the experience with the mother often seems to enhance the experience for both (Bennett et al,

146

1985) and it is common to hear a woman who has recently given birth remark that she 'couldn't have done it without him'.

MEN'S NEEDS IN ANTENATAL CLASSES

The author's own investigation (Nolan, 1994) into what men want from their antenatal classes identified three major areas. (See Box 9.1)

Box 9.1 WHAT MEN WANT FROM ANTENATAL CLASSES

1. Information about labour and how to support partner

- 'To know how to help my partner during labour'
- 'About the different procedures/options available'
- 'To learn as much as possible about what is happening to my partner's body'
- 'Ignorance is NOT bliss!'

2. To understand the effect the baby will have on current lifestyle

- 'How to support my partner in the neonatal period'
- 'To begin to understand what it will be like when the baby is brought home'
- 'The first few weeks of fatherhood'
- 'To be prepared to handle and deal with the baby competently and safely'
- 'The well-being of my partner and myself'

3. A sense of involvement

- 'To share as much as possible the responsibility of the pregnancy'
- 'To learn about my responsibilities before and after the birth'
- 'Understanding and knowledge sufficient for me to play an integral part in the whole process'
- 'To meet others in a similar situation'

Nichols (1993) suggests that antenatal education may not be meeting fathers' needs because it fails to prepare them adequately for the realities of labour:

> Prenatal classes may focus on the positive shared aspects of childbirth, not on experiences that may be stressful or on feelings that may be viewed by fathers as negative. (p 105)

This is in keeping with commentaries provided by other researchers that parents do not want to be patronized by educators offering a watered-down version of what to expect during labour, birth and the early weeks of parenting (see Chapter 1). Nichols (1993) advises:

Presenting a more realistic picture of a woman's discomfort during labor would be useful for first-time fathers who have not experienced labor and delivery. (p 106)

TEACHING APPROACHES

In an address to the Annual General Meeting of the National Childbirth Trust in 1995, Richard Seel, author of *The Uncertain Father* (1987), warned childbirth educators not to treat fathers merely as 'mothers' little helpers'. By this he was suggesting that men are often marginalized in antenatal classes, instructed in what they can do to help their partners during labour and after the birth, but not considered to have needs of their own. Seel's views are borne out by the research of Gottlieb and Pancer (1988) into Lamaze classes:

> *Although the Lamaze method casts the father into the role of a supportive ally vis-a-vis his wife, it does not make any provisions for* him *to receive support either from other fathers or from the whole class. The literature on the transition to parenthood tends to ignore the ways that the father's social network socializes him into the parent role and aids or constrains his strivings to integrate this identity within his marital and work life.* (p 265)

This failure, whilst inexcusable, may be explained by the simple fact that the vast majority of childbirth educators are women. Women educators may need to make a conscious effort to appreciate men's perspective on childbirth and early parenting and to empathize with their experience.

When they are uncertain about how to meet the needs of the men attending their classes, or even what those needs are, the most logical step is to ask the men to speak for themselves. An introductory exercise carried out in single-sex groups to ask men and women what they want from their antenatal classes enables the educator to see where differences in emphasis lie. Comparisons between the two lists may yield some interesting results, although the educator should be aware that men may be so indoctrinated into their role as 'mothers' little helpers' that they fail to consider their own needs as fathers. Difficulty in acknowledging that they have their own emotional involvement in the birth of their child and areas of concern that may be different from those of their partners often reflects men's lack of opportunity to talk about the impact of the pregnancy on their lives and their hopes and fears for the future.

LANGUAGE TO ENSURE EQUAL ACCESS

The childbirth educator demonstrates the extent to which she is committed to the men attending her classes through her use of language. It is easy to fall into the trap of using 'you' to refer to the mothers, and 'the men' or 'the fathers' when addressing the males in the group Relaxation exercises may be unintentionally discriminatory when they refer to the babies '*you* are nourishing in *your* womb' and who are hearing '*your* heartbeat' and thereby fail to acknowledge the fathers' relationship with their unborn children. Similarly, the wording of worksheets should always be checked to ensure that the men are invited to consider issues from their point of view. This means that a question about caesarean sections for small group work could be worded:

> 'Do you want to stay with each other if your baby needs to be born by caesarean?'

rather than:

> 'Do you want your partner to accompany you if your baby needs to be born by caesarean?'

The educator can show in numerous small ways that, when she says 'you', she really means *all* the people attending her class. If she is conducting a labour rehearsal, she asks:

'You've decided that now is the time to go to hospital. How do you feel?' (looking round the group, inviting comments from both the mothers and the fathers).

If it is only the women who tend to respond to open-ended questions, some positive discrimination may be engaged in to draw out the men:

'How do *you* feel, Matt?'

'Would you agree with what Janine has said, Melvyn?'

'Is there an issue here for fathers?'

SINGLE-SEX SMALL GROUP WORK

Single-sex small group work enables men to identify their particular concerns about birth and early parenting, and these may well be different from those of the pregnant women in the class. Men may be more eager than women to project ahead to the time after the birth and to anticipate how their relationship with their partners might change, how they will cope at work after sleepless nights and how they will manage financially. Where pregnant women tend almost exclusively to worry about the well-being of their babies, men worry about both their partners and their babies, making their anxiety at least as great as the mothers', if not greater. (In the author's own survey of 30 expectant fathers (Nolan, 1994), well over half mentioned the health of the mother as being of greater concern to them than the health of their baby.) Small group work which offers men an opportunity to share their worries is invaluable. (See Box 9.2)

If the educator asks one of the men to summarize the key points of their discussion for the whole group, she draws the men's views and feelings to the attention of the women in the class. She may volunteer to type out the strategies the men have devised for coping with anticipated difficulties and distribute copies at the next class.

Handouts are powerful teaching aids because they are a permanent record of the antenatal class's activities and can build up the self-esteem of group members. They boost men's self-esteem when they refer to their needs as individuals as well as the ways in which they can support their partners. Once again, the choice of words and expressions is crucial. (See Handouts 9.1 and 9.2)

TEACHING ABOUT THE FATHER'S ROLE IN LABOUR

It is helpful for childbirth educators to be familiar with some of the research (e.g. Bertsch et al, 1988; Nichols, 1993) that has looked at the roles men adopt during labour. Nichols asked men who had recently been with their partners during labour and birth what they considered were the most helpful things they had done. Forty per cent mentioned small comfort measures such as 'holding her hand' and 'scratching her back'. Respondents also talked about the psychological support they had provided – 'encouragement', 'support' and 'reassurance'. One-fifth of the fathers mentioned the importance of 'just being there' and some referred to communication behaviours such as 'talking to my wife' and 'listening to her'. These responses bear out Bertsch's research, which found that few men were able to adopt the role of 'coach' for which, perhaps, their childbirth educators hoped they had prepared them. Most took on the role of

BOX 9.2 SINGLE-SEX SMALL GROUPS: WORKSHEETS FOR FATHERS

Aim

- to establish a support network for fathers

Learning outcome

- fathers will have identified areas of common and individual concern regarding pregnancy, labour and early parenting

1. Feelings about Pregnancy

How did you feel when you found out that your partner was pregnant?

What have you found the most worrying aspects of the pregnancy?

How do you feel about being present at the birth of your baby?

2. Labour and Birth

What are the three things that most worry you about your partner's labour?

What are the three things you are most looking forward to about being with your partner in labour?

How do you think you will react when your baby is born?

3. After the Birth

What do you think you will find most enjoyable about being a father?

What do you think you will find most difficult?

How will you cope with these difficulties?

What support will you need?

Where will you get the support you need?

'observer' of the labour and confined themselves to 'being there', as mentioned in Nichols' study.

The childbirth educator needs to recognize the fact that many men are unable to provide all the physical or even emotional support that women need during labour; she needs to give permission for the men simply to 'be there'. Whilst there is much talk in childbirth education circles about the importance of not making women feel failures if they choose to have pain relief during labour or to bottle-feed their babies, there is less concern about how men might feel if they have been educated to offer a type of support which, on the day, they find themselves unable to provide. Whenever skills for labour are practised during antenatal classes, the childbirth teacher needs to encourage both the men who are keen to join in with their partners as they try out different positions and breathing patterns *and* those who choose simply to sit near their partners or hold their hands.

HANDOUT 9.1
Checklist for Labour Supporters

P	POSITION	Is your partner changing her position regularly.
		Are you checking that your own position is comfortable if you are massaging her or holding her during contractions?
U	URINATION	Is your partner going to the toilet every hour?
		Are you calling the midwife to be with her from time to time so that you can have a break when you need to?
R	RELAXATION	Is your partner as relaxed as possible?
		Are you as relaxed as possible?
R	RESPIRATION	Is she breathing evenly?
		Is your own breathing calm, your shoulders loose, your face muscles relaxed?
R	REST	Is she taking advantage of the break between contractions?
		Are you refreshing yourself between contractions (having a drink, wiping your face, having a stretch).
R	REASSURANCE	Are you encouraging, praising and talking to your partner?
		Are you asking the midwife for the information you need and seeking support from her?

© Harcourt Brace and Company Limited 1998

HANDOUT 9.2
For Supporters

USEFUL THINGS TO TAKE WITH YOU FOR LABOUR

You need to look after yourself during labour so that you can go on giving your partner the support she needs. Remember that hospitals and especially labour wards tend to be very hot places, so you need to wear cool, comfortable clothing. Even if your baby is being born at home, you will still feel the emotional heat. You also need to have plenty to drink during labour, and to take regular small snacks to keep your energy levels up

You might find the following things helpful to you or your partner during labour:

- Ice-cubes in a wide-topped thermos flask. You could flavour these with fruit juice if you like. They're very refreshing for both of you to suck between contractions

- food to eat during labour – things like nuts, fruit, raisins, chocolate, whatever you think you both might fancy

- woolly socks and a warm shawl or cardigan to wrap your partner in if she suddenly feels cold or shaky

- oil for massaging your partner – almond oil is good, or just an ordinary good-quality vegetable oil from a supermarket

- a sponge or face flannel to wipe your partner's face and your own

- extra pillows (no matter how many the hospital provides, you'll always be able to use more)

- a cassette player and tapes of some favourite music to help you both relax

- food and drink (something special) to celebrate after the birth. Most women are ravenous after they have given birth, and you'll probably feel the same

- small change or a phone card to make telephone calls

- your camera and a film to take pictures of your baby

© Harcourt Brace and Company Limited 1998

GENDER AND LEARNING STYLES

While this book has placed great emphasis on the value of small group work and discussion in antenatal classes as strategies for enabling parents to share their thoughts and feelings and for modelling dependency on peers rather than on professionals, some theorists have suggested that group learning may be more attuned to women's needs than to men's:

> Women have a primary concern with interpersonal relationships, which serve as a key source of their self-identity and personal development. Accordingly, women (are) characterised as more able to learn from one another, or in a collaborative mode, than alone or in a competitive mode. Gender (is) seen as the basis for this preferred learning style. In contrast, men (are) assumed to place more value on autonomy and individual achievement as their source of identity and growth, and thus to be more likely to succeed in autonomous learning situations. (Hayes and Smith, 1994, p 212)

Many educators of adults would agree that men respond well to structured teaching approaches and to class content that is primarily factual. When asked why they have come to antenatal classes, men will often reply that they want 'to find out *what* is going to happen' during labour. Men gain confidence through knowing 'the facts' whereas women, it might be argued, gain confidence from discussing how they might *feel*.

It is not suggested here that one learning mode is more valuable than the other. If people come to classes with different learning styles, whether that difference is based on intellectual ability, life experience or gender, it is the responsibility of the childbirth educator to cater for those differences. Every learner contains within him or herself needs which might be described as 'feminine' and those that might be described as 'masculine'. A rounded learning experience involves engaging in a variety of activities responsive to all aspects of the individual's psyche. Men attending antenatal classes may gain from being encouraged to look at their emotions and to acknowledge their dependency on others, and women from participating in formal learning opportunities which enable knowledge to be absorbed, retained and made available for later use in decision-making.

In an antenatal course for couples, small group work can be balanced by teaching approaches that cater for what might be described as a 'male orientation' towards learning. Acquisition and retention of factual information is made easier if the educator summarizes the key points of her presentations and provides frequent opportunities for people to recap what they have learned. Both men and women will be helped to learn if the educator organizes each class and her entire course in a logical manner so that clients are helped to understand, for example, how labour progresses and what skills might be useful at each stage. Learning about relaxation is facilitated when the educator starts by enabling her group to gain a basic understanding of the contrast between muscles that are tense and those that are relaxed, and then moves on to consider relaxation techniques that seek to influence the body through the mind. Many people may be helped to cope with the challenges of parenting by learning a structured approach to identifying problems, recognizing whose they are and devising strategies for dealing with them.

Quizzes might be considered to represent a 'masculine' competitive approach to learning, but will almost certainly be enjoyed by the whole group. (See Handout 9.3)

HANDOUT 9.3
Babies!

1. How many feeds might your baby need in the first 24 hours of life?

2. How many feeds per day might a breastfed baby need when s/he is 2 weeks old?

3. At what age might you expect your baby to be 'in a routine'?

4. What colour are breastfed babies' nappies?

5. What colour are bottle-fed babies' nappies?

6. How many nappies per week might you use for your baby during the first 3 months of his/her life?

7. What can you do to protect your baby against cot death?

8. What is the minimum age your baby should be before s/he has any solid food?

9. At what age can you give your baby ordinary cow's milk?

10. Do you need to use soap for washing your baby?

11. How often do you need to bath your baby?

12. What diseases can you have your baby immunized against?

© Harcourt Brace and Company Limited 1998

BONDING AND INFANT STIMULATION EXERCISES

Research suggests that men are often better able than their partners to anticipate and plan for the postnatal period (Nolan, 1994). Childbirth educators have a vital role to play in promoting effective and satisfying parenting, and one of the ways of doing this is by bolstering fathers' sense of their importance in their infants' development. There is evidence to suggest that men who are able to attach to their babies during pregnancy and the early neonatal period are better able to interact with their children later on:

> *The overall message is that nurturing and bonding are no longer 'female' experiences but rather responsibilities and joys shared by both parents.* (Peterson and Walls, 1991, p 39)

Fathers can be helped to visualize their infants in the womb during relaxation sessions. It is empowering to share with fathers the research that suggests unborn babies can sense stroking and patting through the abdominal wall and will respond with movement towards the

---

BOX 9.3 INFANT STIMULATION – DISCUSSION POINTS

Touch Infants who have lots of skin-to-skin cuddling with their parents grow and develop faster than those who don't. Stroking, massaging and cuddling a baby are not just an expression of love but nature's way of enabling your baby to grow.

Hearing Babies can recognize their parents' voices from an early age. They enjoy rhythmical music, which is why they find nursery rhymes and lullabies soothing. Talk to your baby in a high-pitched voice with plenty of variation.

Sight Babies prefer black and white for about the first 6 months of their lives because these colours present the greatest possible contrast. They also like to look at their parents' faces and other people's faces. Show your baby his own face in a mirror and draw geometric shapes in black and white on pieces of paper for him to look at.

Smell Babies like sweet smells such as the smell of breast milk or fruit. They also recognize and enjoy the smell of their parents. Putting an item of clothing in the cot, such as a head scarf or cardigan which one parent has worn for a couple of days, will help your baby relax. Taking the baby into the kitchen also provides her with a range of smells to enjoy.

Balance Your baby's middle ear detects changes in position. You can stimulate her sense of movement by rocking her, swinging her, dancing with her and carrying her in a sling. The games fathers often play with their babies – such as bouncing them and throwing them up in the air – are an instinctive response to babies' developmental needs.

(Adapted from Ludington-Hoe, 1985)

---

stimulus (Lux Flanagan, 1996). Fathers are often surprised to learn that it is quite possible to hear their babies' heartbeat, either by putting their ear to the mother's tummy or by using a toilet roll core to focus the sound.

Providing the group with a variety of pictures of newborn babies can facilitate discussion about their individuality. From this point, it is easy to move on to talking about ways of playing with babies which both men and women can enjoy. (See Box 9.3)

It may be that fathers who are aware of the importance of stimulation for their babies' healthy growth and development will participate more actively in the early months of their lives:

> Researchers have stressed the value, for the development of both children and fathers, of having fathers involved not only in the support of the mother and in relating to older children, but also in nurturing young infants. Fathers themselves have desired more active and meaningful participation in the lives of their children. (Notman and Nadelson, 1982, p 132)

Childbirth educators who are skilled in helping their male clients learn in classes can justifiably claim that antenatal education has an influence that persists well beyond labour and birth and contributes to the overall well-being of society through the promotion of good early parenting practices and the integration of the new family unit.

KEY POINTS

1. **Men are often marginalized in antenatal classes, instructed in what they can do to help their partners during labour and after the birth, but not considered to have needs of their own.**

2. **Antenatal education may not be meeting fathers' needs because it fails to prepare them adequately for the *realities* of labour from their point of view.**

3. **Single-sex small group work gives men a chance to identify their particular concerns about birth and early parenting.**

4. **Many men enjoy a structured approach to learning with an emphasis on 'the facts'.**

5. **Men's self-esteem as fathers is enhanced when they understand the role they can play in fostering their infants' development.**

REFERENCES

Bennett A, Hewson D, Booker E and Holliday S (1985) Antenatal preparation and labor support in relation to birth outcomes. *Birth* **12**: 9–16.

Bertsch TD, Nagashima-Whalen L, Dykeman S, Kennell J and McGrath S (1990) Labour support by first time fathers: direct observation with a comparison to experienced doulas. *Journal of Psychosomatic Obstetrics and Gynaecology* **11**: 251–260.

Chapman L (1992) Expectant fathers' roles during labor and birth. *Journal of Obstetric, Gynaecological and Neonatal Nursing* **21**: 114–119.

Duncan S and Markman H (1988) Intervention programs for the transition to parenthood: current status from a prevention perspective. *Pre- and Peri-Natal Psychology Journal* **2**(1): 25–42.

Lux Flanagan G (1996) Beginning life. London: Dorling Kindersley.

Gottlieb BH and Pancer SM (1988) Social networks and the transition to parenthood. In Michaels GY and Goldberg WA (eds) *The Transition to Parenthood: Current Theory and Research*, pp 235–269. New York: Cambridge University Press.

Hayes ER and Smith L (1994) Women in adult education: an analysis of perspectives in major journals. *Adult Education Quarterly* **44**(4): 201–221.

Ludington-Hoe S (1985) *How to Have a Smarter Baby*. New York: Rawson Associates.

Nichols MR (1993) Paternal perspectives of the childbirth experience. *Maternal–Child Nursing Journal* **21**(3): 99–107.

Nolan M (1994) Caring for fathers in antenatal classes. *Modern Midwife* **4**(2): 25–28.

Notman M and Nadelson C (1982) Maternal work and children. In Notman M and Nadelson C (eds) *The Woman Patient, Vol. 2: Concepts of Femininity and the Life Cycle*, pp 121–136. New York: Plenum Press.

Odent M (1994) *Birth Reborn*, 2nd edn. London: Souvenir Press.

Peterson FL and Walls D (1991) Fatherhood preparation during childbirth education. *International Journal of Childbirth Education* **November**: 38–39.

Raphael D (1973) *The Tender Gift: Breastfeeding*. New Jersey: Prentice Hall.

Seel R (1987) *The Uncertain Father*. Bath: Gateway Books.

Sosa R, Kennell J, Klaus M, Robertson S and Urrutia J (1980) The effect of a supportive companion on perinatal problems, length of labor, and mother–infant interaction. *New England Journal of Medicine* **303**: 597–600.

10 Special Parents

Whilst it is entirely legitimate to strive to make classes as excellent as possible for the parents who do attend and who clearly enjoy the kind of learning experiences generally provided by classes, it has to be borne in mind that they reach only a minority of parents (Hancock, 1994; Pugh et al, 1994). Many classes throughout the UK are composed entirely of white middle-class women and their partners who are expecting their first baby. Far less commonly represented are women expecting twins or super-twins, teenage mothers, parents who are about to adopt a baby, disabled parents, parents expecting their second or subsequent child, parents from ethnic minority groups and parents who are unemployed, poor or ill-educated (Sturrock and Johnson, 1990; Young, 1990; Redman et al, 1991; Chadwick, 1994; Meikle et al, 1995). Women who have to spend large parts or the whole of their pregnancy in hospital may miss out on antenatal education entirely. Women who have conceived as a result of infertility treatment may be present at classes, but their very special needs may be unacknowledged.

There is a dearth of research into how antenatal education can be tailored to meet the needs of the special groups mentioned above. The literature concerning classes for special parents is patchy and largely anecdotal. Amongst childbirth educators, there may be very little sharing of experiences about teaching parents with special needs because there is very little experience to be shared.

It is important to acknowledge, therefore, that the ideas this chapter puts forward for reaching parents with special needs are, for the most part, merely ideas and do not have the backing of research. They have been gleaned from a few educators who are experienced in working with non-traditional groups of antenatal class attenders. There is a great need for more research into how antenatal education can be made more attractive to a wider audience. Until that is available, it is important for childbirth educators to seize every opportunity to observe classes for parents with special needs, to talk to the people running them and to start to draw together ideas for making childbirth education truly accessible to every parent.

REACHING LOW-INCOME PARENTS

Poverty is a major cause of neonatal mortality. Poor eating habits may be coupled with heavy dependency on smoking and alcohol, and thereby place the health of the mother and her baby in jeopardy. Underprivileged women are more likely to give birth to premature babies, more likely to give birth to babies who are small for dates, more likely to have babies who are ill at birth and more likely to have babies who die at or around birth (Chadwick, 1994).

Women on a low income do not, however, usually attend antenatal classes, either those provided by lay organizations such as the National Childbirth Trust and the Active Birth Centre or those offered at hospitals and clinics. Attracting this group of women and their families to classes requires a new approach. The Florida Outreach Childbirth Education Project may provide a useful model (Jeffers, 1992).

This project was set up as a result of a survey in the late 1980s which revealed that antenatal classes provided in Florida were not accessible to low-income, low-literacy families, that classes were often run by health professionals who were not trained as educators and who did not perceive childbirth education to be a priority in an area of significant social disadvantage, and that there was little funding available for extending the scope or quality of classes.

The strategies adopted to address this situation were to recruit a large number of childbirth educators from the private sector and to improve the training of health professionals in antenatal education. Regional coordinators were appointed to expand the childbirth education programme into new areas and different communities, and health professionals collaborated with a variety of social care and charitable agencies in order to plan, develop, implement and evaluate outreach programmes. Funding was sought from charities, community education programmes, hospitals and public health authorities. Classes were conducted primarily in adult and community education centres and were advertised widely using well designed, colourful and easy-to-read posters.

Teaching goals in relation to antenatal education for disadvantaged families were clearly specified so that all educators were clear about what it was they were hoping to achieve. (See Box 10.1)

The content of classes was based on the needs identified by the parents themselves. Teaching methods included low-literacy written materials, and feedback was obtained from clients using questionnaires specially designed for adults with low-literacy skills.

The project has been extremely successful as measured by the number of very low-income parents who attend antenatal classes in Florida each year. Whilst the organization of health care in the United States is quite different from that in the UK, this should not prevent us from being open to those elements of the Florida programme that could be transposed into the UK arena. The problem of reaching parents from social classes III(M), IV and V has been with us for many years and demands innovative schemes in order to address it.

REACHING PARENTS FROM ETHNIC MINORITIES

Montgomery (1991) writes poignantly of the nightmare endured by women who do not speak English and/or whose cultural needs around birth are not understood by health professionals:

> *Imagine you have just given birth. You are in a foreign country. The health care providers speak a language unknown to you. The birthing practices are unfamiliar and frightening. You are confused and intimidated by the hustle and bustle going on all around you. Although you understand very little about the procedures, you quietly go*

BOX 10.1 TEACHING GOALS: THE FLORIDA OUTREACH CHILDBIRTH EDUCATION PROGRAM

1. To stimulate parents to participate in adult education programmes to further their education, thus enabling them to create a learning environment in their own homes.

2. To increase participants' understanding in the areas of good health, fetal development, preparation for labour and birth, family planning, child care and parenting.

3. To help participants become aware of the consequences of their behaviours and of the range of their choices.

4. To offer participants positive reinforcements of problem-solving skills in an accepting environment.

5. To influence participants to choose habits that support healthy lifestyle and positive parenting behaviours.

6. To increase the likelihood of participants having the most positive birth experiences by building confidence in their own capabilities.

(From Jeffers, 1992)

---

along with them because you have heard that it is risky to question the authorities. You could get into trouble. They might even take your baby away from you.

Yes, it's been a bizarre experience to say the least, but your baby is here at last. The baby you have waited for and loved while you carried him is here and he's perfect. Wait a minute! Something is terribly wrong! They've just brought your baby back into the room and he is dressed in funeral clothes. Is your baby going to die? Why is everyone so unconcerned? Your baby is dying and no one seems to care! (Montgomery, 1991)

Montgomery points out that the colour white, often chosen in the West for clothes and blankets for new babies, is viewed by many people from South-East Asian cultures as the colour of mourning. Cultural sensitivity must be the foundation of any educational programme for people from ethnic minority groups. Childbirth educators need to familiarize themselves with the cultural beliefs and practices of their target groups and be prepared to have their own ideas about birthing and childrearing challenged. Cultural sensitivity is most easily and fully achieved when educators are recruited from the ethnic group itself. Such educators are seen as role models by the parents whom they teach in a way that women who are from a different racial or cultural group are not. Flexibility in the timing of classes may be critical. Asian women often have domestic responsibilities which prevent them from attending classes held at times when they are preparing meals. Transportation can be a problem. A successful parentcraft programme for Asian women in Preston in the north-west of England is based on providing a dedicated minibus service to collect the women booked for classes from their homes (Edwards, 1995). The link-worker travels on the bus and knocks at each woman's door. Asian women may find it easier to gain permission from their mother-in-law to attend classes if the mother-in-law is invited to attend as well.

It is easy to assume that Asian women are always part of an extended family which includes experienced mothers who will help them through the early postnatal weeks. This may not be the case, and Asian women, like white women, often express a desire to learn basic babycare skills such as nappy changing, bathing, soothing and how to put a baby down to sleep. Nor do ethnic women necessarily know all about breastfeeding. There may be as much wrong information about infant feeding and weaning held within a minority ethnic group as within the dominant culture, and the childbirth educator must work in the usual way to find out what parents already know, correct any misinformation and build on their existing skills and under-standing to foster good infant-feeding practices.

When a childbirth educator and link-worker or translator are running classes together, communication beforehand about the material to be covered during the session, the kind of discussion the educator wants to promote, and the practical work to be undertaken is essential. The educator needs to express herself clearly and concisely in class and be able to hold on to her train of thought during the intervals when the link-worker is translating. She also needs to be able to wait patiently and allow discussion to happen, handing control of the class over to the women even in a situation where she does not know what they are saying to one another. The link-worker needs to be able to listen carefully and pick out and feed back to the educator the issues that she knows the educator will want to develop more fully.

A serious difficulty facing childbirth educators working with ethnic women is the lack of suitable material written in the women's own languages. A second-best option is to give class attenders leaflets written in English and to invite them to ask a friend or relative to translate for them. It is also very difficult to find visual aids and videos that portray non-Caucasian babies and families. Childbirth educators can lobby suppliers of teaching aids to meet this need and themselves build up a library of pictures appropriate for classes attended by women and their supporters from a variety of cultures. An enterprising group of midwives involved in parent-craft education in Bradford worked with a local video production company to make videos in Urdu and Bengali which could be used in classes for Asian women:

> We hope that our videos present a positive image of pregnancy and childbirth for Asian women and that they will stimulate discussion. Our aim is to meet the identified need for more relevant parent education which will enable Pakistani and Bangladeshi women in Bradford and elsewhere to make appropriate choices and become active partners in care. (Walker and Pollard, 1995, p 23)

There is considerable scope for more initiatives of this kind.

Finally, it should be observed that there is very little research into whether people from different racial groups have the same learning styles. What has been written about adult education has been written by white researchers and based on groups made up of white learners. Within psychology, little attention is paid to normal *women* let alone normal black women. Understanding of the educational needs of black people, and especially black women, is minimal (A. Phoenix, speaking on Radio 4, 2 June 1996).

REACHING HOSPITALIZED WOMEN

Whilst medical care for the pregnant woman at high risk has improved immeasurably over the last quarter century, as has treatment for very sick and premature babies, the educational needs of the mother who is compelled to spend long periods of her pregnancy in hospital have been very much overlooked.

Whilst hospitalized women may have many opportunities to receive education on a one-to-one basis from midwives, their need for educational affiliation, especially with women in similar circumstances, remains paramount. In addition, their partners need to share the considerable anxiety associated with at-risk pregnancies with others who are shouldering the same burden.

The aims of classes for hospitalized high-risk women are (Avery and McKenzie, 1987):

- to decrease anxiety

- to enhance each woman's relationship with her unborn baby

- to enable partners to have a better understanding of each other's needs

Whilst much of the content of classes will be similar to that provided for women experiencing normal pregnancies, some topics need special attention.

Relaxation Techniques

Relaxation techniques are particularly important because they can enable a woman at high risk to manage her fears and conserve her energy for her own well-being and that of her baby, not only during labour but also during the long weeks of pregnancy.

Signs of Pre-term Labour

Women having pregnancy difficulties need to be able to recognize the signs of pre-term labour and know what action they should take if labour starts during weekend leave or after they have been discharged.

Caesarean Section

Because of the increased likelihood of at risk women needing to give birth by caesarean section, antenatal education should cover this topic in depth, with an emphasis on helping women to think about the support they will need after they leave hospital.

Special Care

Women at high risk and their partners should have the chance to discuss with each other the support they will need after the birth if their babies have medical problems.

Bonding

Women whose pregnancies are at risk may protect themselves from hurt by distancing themselves emotionally from the babies they are carrying. Whereas most women experiencing normal pregnancy establish a close bond with their unborn babies, talk to them in the womb and make extensive preparations for their arrival, high-risk women may choose to make no preparations, refuse to consider names, and avoid looking at or touching their bellies. These women need time to talk about their feelings towards their babies and to be reassured that ambiguous or even hostile feelings are normal and not shameful. Childbirth educators can show the mother whose pregnancy is at risk how to massage her baby in utero by lightly stroking her stomach, and encourage her to become aware of how her baby is lying and of his patterns of waking and sleeping. If the baby dies, the mother will find it easier to grieve if she has previously allowed herself to create an identity for her baby (Mander, 1994).

Infant Feeding

Bonding with a small, sickly, premature infant can be greatly helped if the mother is able to provide her own milk for her child. Antenatal classes for hospitalized women should therefore include discussion and information about how women can express their milk to tube-feed their babies, about cup feeding and about putting very small babies to the breast.

Reaching Parents With Disabilities

Many people who are able bodied find themselves uncomfortable in the presence of someone who has a disability. They fear causing offence, and are not sure how much assistance to offer or to what extent the disabled person should be treated 'differently'. Educators need to explore their own prejudices around disability before attempting to deliver a sensitive and useful service to parents with disabilities. Typical stereotypes imposed by able-bodied people include:

- Disabled people don't have normal intelligence.

- Disabled people are dependent.

- A disabled person is an ill person.

- All disabled women have to give birth by caesarean section.

- The child of a disabled person is at risk.

- A disabled person cannot be a proper parent.

(based on Campion, 1990)

A more accurate stereotype might be that disabled couples who choose to become parents are likely to have given far greater thought to their decision than the majority of able-bodied people who embark on a pregnancy. They cannot escape acknowledging the difficulties they face both in terms of looking after their children and in terms of combating and helping their children to combat hostile social attitudes.

Once the childbirth educator knows that a disabled woman is attending her classes, she needs to make a point of contacting her beforehand to ask what facilities she needs and what topics she is particularly interested in. As much as able-bodied people, disabled people like to be independent and the only way in which the educator can find out what help the disabled woman or couple needs, what practical work they can participate in and what is not possible for them, is by asking.

Most disabled people like to attend ordinary antenatal classes alongside able-bodied parents rather than being singled out for one-to-one attention from the midwife or childbirth educator. The educator has to try to strike a balance between adapting the skills parents are learning in her classes to the needs of the disabled couple and not drawing attention to the couple all the time as a 'special case'.

Aims in relation to antenatal classes for disabled women were summarized by Elaine Carty and Tali Conine in their address in May 1993 to the International Confederation of Midwives:

It is anticipated that a successful program could potentially result in:

- *well-informed women who are in control over a major lifestyle decision*

- *mothers whose skills are enhanced to their maximum potential through aids, adaptations and assistance to give independent and safe care to their infants and toddlers*

- *women whose self-esteem is enhanced through confidence in their abilities to do what 'normal' women do*

- *ultimately a decrease in the use of medical and social services by women with disabilities for their parenting and child care needs.* (Carty and Conine, 1993)

The following learning opportunities have been found by disabled parents to be helpful:

- a guided tour round the hospital where their baby is to be born, to familiarize themselves with the environment and to talk to staff about their needs. It may fall to the childbirth educator to arrange such a visit at a time when staff are not too busy.

- being put in touch with other parents who have the same disability

- being introduced to organizers of local mother and baby groups – isolation postnatally is a real problem for disabled parents

- being put in touch with organizations with specialist knowledge of disability and parenting. Research suggests that disabled women rely more on lay sources for guidance about babycare and equipment than they do on health professionals

- having individual attention both antenatally and postnatally to learn about breast-feeding. Bottle-feeding may be dangerous for women who have difficulty sterilizing bottles because of sight impairment or problems using their hands

- pictures of disabled parents and their children

(McEwan Carty et al, 1990)

REACHING PARENTS WHO ARE DEAF

If a deaf woman or couple choose to come to antenatal classes with parents who have normal hearing, it is likely that they will be accompanied by an interpreter. The childbirth educator is, however, providing learning opportunities for the parents and not their interpreter, and should address all her remarks to them. If the parents are unaccompanied by an interpreter, the educator needs to find out whether they can lip-read or whether they communicate through writing. If they lip-read, it is important for the educator to position herself so that her face can be seen clearly. Even someone who is skilled at lip-reading can interpret only about 25% of what is being said, and the educator must check that parents have understood the information being given or the work the class is doing. People who have been deaf from birth or early childhood may have limited reading skills, although they are of normal intelligence. The childbirth educator needs therefore to ensure that any handouts she uses are written at basic literacy level. When displaying visual aids, she needs to take into account that deaf people cannot look at a picture and lip-read or observe someone who is signing all at the same time. They need time to look at the picture or teaching aid and then back to the educator or signer.

REACHING PARENTS WHO ARE BLIND OR PARTIALLY SIGHTED

People who are blind learn about the world through listening and touching. The challenge to childbirth educators is therefore to present information with maximum clarity and to devise or identify teaching aids that the blind woman or couple can handle to enhance their learning. Partially sighted parents may be able to see charts or read what is written on a flipchart if the writing is in large, bold letters with maximum contrast (black on white) between letter colour and background paper. A totally blind woman can understand how her baby will be born if the educator gives her a model pelvis and guides her hands down through the cavity and outlet, helping her to feel the important landmarks. Even more than normally sighted parents, a couple who are blind will want to gain confidence in babycare skills and are likely to appreciate repeated opportunities to practise changing and bathing a doll or baby.

REACHING PARENTS WHO HAVE LIMITED MOBILITY OR WHO ARE WHEELCHAIR USERS

Antenatal classes should be held at venues that are fully accessible to every parent who wishes to attend. For disabled parents who are wheelchair users, accessibility means wide doorways, a ground floor classroom or one that can be reached by a large and well maintained lift, and specially adapted toilets. A mother who has arthritis or a condition that makes walking difficult will see long flights of stairs and poorly lit corridors as barriers to her attendance. The chairs provided at classes need to be at the right height and sufficiently firm to enable a woman with mobility difficulties to sit down and get up again easily.

Many people who are wheelchair users consider their wheelchair as an extension of their own bodies and it is therefore highly inappropriate for the childbirth educator to lean on the back of the chair or to move it without seeking permission beforehand.

REACHING PARENTS WHO ARE EXPECTING TWINS

Many antenatal classes will include parents who are expecting twins. To cater for their needs, the childbirth educator needs to ensure that the language she uses and the images of birth and parenting she conveys through visual aids embrace the experience of the woman who will be delivering two babies and have two babies to care for. Relaxation sessions that focus on imagining life after birth, for example, must create a picture to which parents expecting twins can relate as well as those expecting a single baby.

While the woman who is expecting twins will probably enjoy the extra interest her situation attracts, she may find it hard to obtain the information and acquire the skills that she needs to help her through the transition to parenthood. Just as the childbirth educator strives to give parents of singletons a realistic idea of what labour and early parenting are like, she needs to do the same for those who are expecting twins. Although a twin pregnancy is a perfectly normal biological occurrence, it is known to be associated with a higher risk of pregnancy complications, with interventions during labour (induction, epidural anaesthesia, caesarean section) and with postnatal unhappiness and illness afterwards (Thorpe et al, 1991). Classes that include parents of twins therefore need to cover certain issues particularly thoroughly:

- pre-eclampsia – warning signs
- interventions during labour
- Special Care Baby Unit
- physical recovery of the mother postnatally
- postnatal mental health

The woman who is expecting twins may be particularly concerned about the extent to which she will be in control of the care she receives during labour. There is scope for the childbirth educator to talk to her and her partner individually about how their babies will be born. Their coping skills will be enhanced if they know in advance that there are likely to be many more people in the delivery room than usual, and that the babies may be taken to Special Care to be observed for a while.

Twin babies are more likely to die at or around birth than single babies. Most parents expecting twins are very aware of this and the normal fears that occasionally overshadow the pregnancies of couples expecting one baby – 'Will our baby be all right? Will our baby be stillborn? How can we protect our baby against cot death?' – will be more prominent in the minds of parents expecting twins. This makes the subject of bereavement both very important for the childbirth educator to raise and very difficult. Sources of support for parents who lose one twin are scarce because there is a tendency for people to assume that the living baby 'makes up' for the dead one. The loss of a baby is no less a loss because he or she was a twin. If both babies die, parents may be made to think that they should feel the tragedy less because their pregnancy was in some way not quite normal. The childbirth educator needs to be able to acknowledge during her classes that babies do die and to help group members think through the grieving process. Should anyone in the group, be it the parents of twins or of a single baby, subsequently experience a birth loss, the educator has, by virtue of having discussed bereavement during her classes, made herself approachable as a source of support.

Helping parents of twins to anticipate postnatal life is a major concern of antenatal education. This means ensuring that there are many learning opportunities that enable them to consider how their lifestyles will change after their babies are born and to plan in advance. Expectant parents of twins need to recognize that they will probably have less time for cuddling their babies than parents who have only one infant to look after and that their decision about infant feeding may need to take this into account. Breastfeeding allows the mother to feed both her babies at once and ensures that she makes time on multiple occasions every day for holding her babies closely. There are, however, disadvantages: the mother may find that her life is a constant round of feeding babies, that she becomes excessively tired and that her opportunities to go out and meet other mothers are reduced because it is hard to feed two babies discreetly in public. The childbirth educator can arrange for the parents expecting twins to meet another couple whose babies are a few months old to discuss with them how they have coped with feeding and the other practical arrangements necessary for looking after two babies. Such a meeting offers the expectant father a rare opportunity to talk to another man about the role he has played since the birth of his babies and to think ahead to how he himself can integrate work and home in a situation where his partner is likely to be highly dependent on his assistance. Hay et al (1990) found that the extent to which the father gives practical help and emotional support to the mother during the first year of twin babies' lives has a significant impact on her mental health.

Including parents of twins in mainstream antenatal classes not only integrates them into 'normal' parental life, but also gives them the benefit of the objectivity that those not in their situation can provide. Issues such as how to establish the individuality of twins, choosing names, whether the babies should be dressed the same and how to ensure each child receives individual attention will be fascinating to all pregnant parents. Opportunities for individual couples to work together during classes enable the parents expecting twins to reflect privately on how information shared or given, issues raised during discussion and practical skills relate to their own situation.

The woman expecting twins will almost certainly have been repeatedly exposed to 'rather you than me' remarks long before she gets to antenatal classes. If people are told sufficiently frequently that they are likely to find caring for twins a nightmare, they almost certainly will. It is important for the childbirth educator to try to strike a balance between a realistic appraisal of the amount of hard work involved in caring for two babies and an acknowledgment of the particular pleasures that watching twins growing up together and interacting with each other can bring. She needs to recognize and help the parents expecting twins to understand that the relationship they will have with their babies will be different from the relationship between parents and one baby:

Other parents might have time to show their babies a book, or take them for walks, but I hardly had time to smile at them. If one was being quiet, I'd rejoice because it meant

that I could change the other one's nappy in peace. Most of the time, though, in those first few months, I felt as if I was listening to a constant grizzle, because – except when it came to feeding – whatever I was giving one, it meant I wasn't giving it to the other.
(McGrail, 1996, p 4)

The task of the childbirth educator is to help expectant parents of twins identify coping strategies and sources of support that will enable them to gain as much satisfaction as possible from the early months and years of parenting. Ensuring that parents of twins know about the Twins and Multiple Births Association and the Multiple Births Foundation, and providing them with contact numbers, is an important detail of the educator's work.

Reaching Parents Who Are Adopting a Baby

Adoption is a cure for childlessness, not for infertility; it means acknowledging that the baby who has arrived is not the couple's own baby, but someone else's. The placement of a baby heralds the end of what is likely to have been a long struggle for the woman or couple to be accepted as adoptive parents. There can be a profound sense of anticlimax when the months, perhaps years, of waiting for a baby to become available are finally over. For the couple whose 'pregnancy' has been open-ended rather than limited to 9 months, the sudden transition to parenthood and caring for a baby full-time can come as a great shock.

Childbirth educators need to be aware that there is still considerable hostility against adoption – and even revulsion. The adoptive parents are likely to have to deal with questions such as: 'Are you sure you can love somebody else's child?' 'How do you know that the baby hasn't got bad blood in him?' 'Of course, you're not her *real* parents.' The crisis of self-confidence that any infertile couple has already gone through may be exacerbated by the doubts of others regarding their ability to parent and love the baby placed with them.

The central task of the childbirth educator is therefore to boost the confidence of the couple who are waiting to have a baby placed with them. They may need considerable reassurance that they can easily acquire the skills necessary to care for a baby and that they have all the normal human resources to nurture a baby emotionally. Reassurance needs to be backed up with practical skills-based antenatal education so that the adoptive parents have multiple opportunities to learn how to care for a baby – how to change nappies, how to bathe, feed and wean their baby, how to recognize signs of illness, and how to cuddle and interact with their baby. Discussion of baby equipment and clothes is important.

The educator needs to ensure that any unintentionally insensitive remarks made by other people in the antenatal group are balanced by her own positive handling of the couple's situation. In practice, parents attending antenatal classes are usually extremely sensitive to each other's needs and the adoptive couple benefits greatly from being part of a mainstream group. The childbirth educator may need to restructure her course if the adoptive couple chooses only to attend classes dealing with postnatal issues so that labour and birth are covered with the rest of the group in their absence.

Adoptive parents need the chance to discuss and learn about postnatal illness in antenatal classes. They are at least as vulnerable as other couples to postnatal unhappiness, which is often linked to:

the tendency on the part of adoptive parents to feel that they must be perfect parents. This tendency has several sources. The obvious one is the special pressure to do well with a child brought into the world by others . . . They, unlike biological parents, must demonstrate . . . that they will be good parents. (Hartman and Laird, 1990, p 235)

Whilst it is likely that their social worker will have put them in touch with post-adoption support groups, adoptive parents will also benefit from being referred by their childbirth educator to a parent and baby group or National Childbirth Trust open house where they can put the joys and difficulties they are experiencing with their baby into the context of normal everyday parenting.

There are those who would argue that the disruption caused in even a small baby's life by being taken away from her natural mother and placed with another woman is immense (Newton Verrier, 1994). The severing of the biological link deprives the baby of the voice, the smell and the touch of the person whose daily rhythms she has become accustomed to since conception. Her need for security is likely to be every bit as great as that of her adoptive parents. The childbirth educator can discuss with the woman or couple waiting to have a baby placed with them ways in which babies are helped to feel secure, such as through skin-to-skin contact, being carried in a sling, and co-sleeping if neither parent is a smoker. Adoptive parents may be more than usually anxious about the growth of their baby and will appreciate learning about developmental milestones and the wide variation in the time it takes individual babies to reach these.

An adoptive mother may believe that breastfeeding will enable her to bond more effectively with her baby, and the childbirth educator should be prepared to discuss with her how this might be achieved. Whilst it is possible for a woman to breastfeed even if she has never been pregnant, she needs to understand the amount of time and commitment she will need to initiate and sustain lactation, and to be prepared for the likelihood that she will be able to meet only some of her baby's feeding requirements. The childbirth educator should refer her to a midwife or breastfeeding counsellor from La Leche League or the National Childbirth Trust with relevant experience and, ideally, put the adoptive mother in contact with a woman who has been successful in initiating lactation in similar circumstances.

Although they may have longed for a baby of their own for many frustrating years, adoptive couples often find, as ordinary parents do, that it takes time for them to feel love for their baby. Antenatal classes can facilitate discussion about patterns of bonding and how falling in love with a baby may be instantaneous – just as some couples fall in love at first sight – or a more gradual process which takes months and even years. Adoptive parents need reassurance that, whatever their feelings when a baby is placed with them, those feelings are as 'right' as anyone else's. By giving them 'permission' to experience the joys and insecurities of parenting to the full, the childbirth educator helps the adoptive woman or couple to grow in confidence in the very special role they have taken on as parents to a baby who might not otherwise have had the benefits of a loving family in which to grow up.

REACHING VERY YOUNG PARENTS

As with all minority groups, teenage mothers are often the victims of stereotyping. Contrary to popular belief, they are not:

- all unmarried
- all unsupported
- all from a background of abuse
- all mentally frail
- all interested in epidurals for their labours

- all determined to bottle-feed their babies

- all incompetent as women and mothers

What is stereotypical is the way in which young mothers are treated by older adults with whom they come into contact. Young pregnant women may find that they are not given explanations by professionals about the care they are receiving or the plans that are being made for them. They may be made to feel stupid and ashamed of themselves and treated with coldness if not outright hostility.

It is a mistake to think that all young mothers are pregnant by accident. Some have made a considered decision to become pregnant and some do not see teenage pregnancy as undesirable. Those who come from a background of deprivation may choose pregnancy as a means of establishing a family separate from the one that has failed them and in which they can find and give love. Some, being the daughters of women who themselves became pregnant at a young age, are adhering to a model of early childbearing. Society chooses to put young mothers in an invidious position by denying them the financial and emotional support provided for other women whom it deems as coming to motherhood at a more appropriate age.

The aims of childbirth education for young mothers is to build up their confidence and sense of achievement, and thereby safeguard the well-being of their children. The Director of a Young Women's Christian Association 'Pregnant Teen/Teen Mothers' programme states the ethos of all those providing services for teen parents as follows:

> We believe that when these young parents feel fulfilled themselves, they can be better parents. (quoted in Hudson and Ineichen, 1994, p 198)

Young pregnant women are likely to feel more secure and therefore enabled to learn more effectively if they attend antenatal classes with a peer group. Their childbirth education may need to be broader than the usual curriculum and include planning and costing meals, prioritizing financially for essential babycare items, healthy lifestyles and how to access support services. Young mothers-to-be may require information and guidance to help them find training opportunities, enter the job market or complete their education after the birth of their babies if that is what they wish to do.

Whilst there is no case for patronizing teenage mothers or for trying to exercise a parental-type control over them, there is room for sensitive and responsive 'mothering' on the part of the childbirth educator to boost their self-esteem and enable them to make a secure and confident transition to parenthood. Some innovative schemes have obtained funding from local authorities and health trusts to provide full-time pregnancy education for young women during the entire period of their pregnancies (Nolan, 1996). Postnatal education for young women is almost non-existent and childbirth educators should consider this an area ripe for development.

REACHING SINGLE MOTHERS

Stereotypes of single mothers suggest that they are always young and poor; of course, they may be neither. There are many reasons why a woman embarks on motherhood as a single person. She may have experienced the breakdown of a short or long-term relationship as a result of her pregnancy or since her pregnancy. She may have made a deliberate choice to become a single mother and her baby may be the result of IVF or of her own deliberate effort to become pregnant by a man with whom she did not wish to share a committed relationship. She may have been widowed since becoming pregnant or have become pregnant accidentally and decided to keep her baby.

Single women may be quite at ease attending classes for couples, appreciating the contributions made by the men and preferring the particular kind of companionship available in a mixed group, or they may want to attend women only classes. Either way, the educator needs to ensure that her choice of words never implies that every woman has a partner or that every woman will be supported in labour by the father of her child. A single woman may need help to think through her options regarding support in labour; she may be unaware that it is possible for her to choose to have her sister or her mother or female friend or a male friend who is not the baby's father with her when she gives birth. The educator needs to think about how she will respond if a single woman asks her to be her labour companion – a not uncommon situation. Can she promise to be available for the woman at whatever time of the day or night she might call upon her? If the answer is no, it is better to say 'no' rather than run the risk of letting the woman down just when she is at her most vulnerable in early labour.

Facilitating practical work on self-help skills for labour is a particular challenge for the childbirth educator whose group includes a single woman – but an excellent opportunity for the educator to think about how she can help prepare a woman to cope on her own in labour if she has to. The educator can choose to work with the woman when the group is practising self-help skills, but the woman also needs to learn how to put the skills into practice on her own.

A single woman will need the time and opportunity to think about where her support will come from after her baby is born. If she is part of an antenatal group that has been helped to develop from a group of individuals who have nothing in common except their pregnancy to a group whose members are interested in and care for each other, she is likely to find that other people in the group will, very probably, offer to support her. The childbirth educator's task is to ensure that discussion of postnatal life embraces the particular needs of the woman who will not have a partner with whom to share the excitement and strain of the first months of parenting.

REACHING LESBIAN PARENTS

As more and more gay people seek to create families, it is likely that childbirth educators will increasingly find themselves welcoming lesbian parents to their antenatal classes. The decision about whether these couples should attend women-only classes or couples classes is a decision for the couples themselves, as is the decision about how much to tell the other parents in the group about their relationship. Some lesbian parents will choose to allow class members to presume that the non-pregnant partner is simply acting as a supporter to the pregnant woman; some are confident in talking openly about their sexuality. Whilst other parents may be shocked, the educator's own acceptance of the couple will set the pattern for making the couple welcome. The educator may be helped to cope with her own possible nervousness about including a lesbian couple if she remembers that, first and foremost, they are people making the transition to parenthood. Their need is exactly the same as that of other parents in her group, namely to prepare themselves for labour, birth and early parenting. If lesbian parents are excluded from parent groups during their pregnancy, they may find it harder to integrate themselves later when to do so is critical for their child, for example when the child is ready to go to school.

There is no need for the educator to avoid single-sex small group work; the non-pregnant partner in the lesbian couple can make her own decision about whether to join the women or the men. If she joins the male group, her ability as a woman to talk about her feelings may enable the men to think about emotional areas that they would otherwise have difficulty exploring (Pattberg, 1997). The educator has to be careful to monitor her use of language: 'fathers', 'men' and 'dads' need to be avoided. If she wants to distinguish between mothers and fathers in a way that is sensitive to the situation of every couple in her class, she needs to refer to 'pregnant women' and 'partners'.

Once it is known that lesbian couples are accepted and included at a particular educator's classes, it is likely that more will come to her. She is then in a position to establish a network of lesbian parents whom she has put in touch with each other. Pregnant couples will benefit from the experience and support of other lesbian couples who have successfully made the transition to parenthood.

REACHING PARENTS EXPECTING THEIR SECOND OR SUBSEQUENT BABY

Whilst the presence in an antenatal group of a woman or couple expecting their second baby is a great asset to the childbirth educator who can draw on their experience to add realism to her classes, the needs of the couple themselves should not be overlooked and may be slightly different from those of parents who are expecting their first babies. Antenatal education for second-time parenthood focuses on two important areas:

1. debriefing previous experiences of labour, birth and early parenting

2. how to integrate a second or subsequent child into the family

To enter into a second labour with confidence, parents need to have reflected on and, if necessary, been helped to understand what happened during their first. Similarly, experiences of infant feeding need to be revisited to enable the couple to make a considered choice about feeding their second baby. The questions that remained unanswered when the woman left hospital after having her first baby often become important only when she is expecting her next. A good first birth experience lends the parents confidence for the second time round, but a poor first experience may undermine the couple's confidence in their ability to give birth.

Often, listening to experienced parents talk about their previous labours and the early weeks of their children's lives is invaluable in increasing the insight of parents who are expecting their first babies. However, childbirth educators need to assess whether second-time parents need more time to debrief than is available in class, and the extent to which first-time parents are benefiting from listening to them. It may be appropriate for the educator to offer time outside the class for parents to talk at length about their previous births.

Parents who are expecting their first baby are often acute observers of parenting styles and of interactions between parents and children and between individual children. Small group work which invites both first- and second-time parents to identify strategies for integrating a new baby into a family that already includes children can be very productive. The first-time parents have the chance to project ahead to what may well be their own situation in a few years' time and feel valued when asked to help more experienced parents.

REACHING PARENTS WITH LEARNING DIFFICULTIES

The stigma that still attaches to people with physical disabilities is perhaps endured to an even greater degree by people with learning difficulties. There is a huge range of learning difficulties and, whilst people who are severely disabled rarely have children, those with mild or moderate degrees of learning disability may actively choose to do so, or simply become pregnant through enjoying a normal, healthy sex life.

The antenatal education of women with learning difficulties ideally needs to start well before they are likely to become pregnant. Education does not aim to persuade these women that they should not have babies, but to help them understand the practical and emotional implications of parenting. If they have received pre-conception education, women with learning difficulties are far more likely to recognize that they are pregnant should pregnancy occur and to present themselves early for care. Women who have had no education about their sexuality and about childbearing may well not attend for antenatal care out of fear that they will be 'punished' for becoming pregnant and their baby taken away from them.

Childbirth educators who welcome women with learning difficulties into their classes are making a great contribution towards boosting their self-esteem. Whether educators are working with these women in an antenatal class or on a one-to-one basis, certain teaching approaches are likely to be fruitful:

> Within the parenthood group, attempts need to be made to present information clearly and visually – other women may benefit too! It can be helpful to tape-record the class, so that the woman can take it home to listen to again. In this way, important information isn't lost or forgotten, and it gives the woman a chance to formulate her own questions if she doesn't understand something. No one with learning disabilities wants attention drawn to them because of their disability, so the answering of seemingly obvious or repetitive questions needs to be carried out respectfully, valuing the woman, and giving the required information. (Dixon, 1996, p 9)

Sometimes women with learning difficulties and their partners are invited to attend antenatal classes arranged for very young parents. This is far from ideal. Both groups tend to feel undervalued and the kind of learning opportunities that are appropriate for teenage parents are not necessarily appropriate for people whose learning difficulties require the educator to spend a lot of time presenting information, reviewing it, consolidating it and ensuring that it has been understood.

It is well known that those who have been fortunate enough to receive good parenting when they were children often make the transition to parenthood more easily than those who have not. Many people with learning difficulties have been abused as children (M.J. Campion, personal communication, 1996) and thus preparing them to become parents is a special challenge for educators. Survivors benefit from establishing a close relationship with one or two carers who provide all their educational and clinical care, preferably in a non-threatening environment away from the hospital or surgery. However, a support network is also essential and the educator needs to ensure that the woman or couple has access to groups of other parents with learning difficulties or parent groups in the community where they will be made welcome.

Parents with learning difficulties are no different from those with normal intelligence in their need for antenatal education that responds to their particular learning style and for support that continues into the postnatal period. When appropriate learning opportunities are made available and there is continuity of care from pre-conception to the postnatal period, the outlook for parents with learning difficulties is very good. It is surely more sensible to invest in the education and support of these parents so that they are enabled to take responsibility for their baby than to incur the enormous expense of having to take the child into care at a later stage if things go wrong.

SUMMARY

The main challenge facing childbirth educators who want to meet the educational needs of special groups of parents is to attract them to classes in the first place. Parents' reluctance to attend may be directly correlated to the amount of prejudice they have already encountered within the health and social care systems or which they fear they may encounter. Childbirth educators need to ensure that they have thoroughly explored and understood their own prejudices and that the language, images, teaching aids and teaching strategies they are using in classes reflect their awareness of the importance of providing equal opportunities for all parents.

The debate about whether it is better to provide education for parents with particular needs in groups separate from mainstream classes is ongoing. Enabling these parents to learn alongside 'regular' class attenders makes the important and democratic point that the transition to parenthood is an experience with common features no matter what the parents' race, culture, sexuality, religion, economic status, physical or mental abilities, but there is also a case for providing separate classes which allow the educator to tailor learning opportunities to the needs of certain identified groups of parents. It may be easier to attract parents with special needs into antenatal education if they are able to be part of a peer group where they feel that their concerns will be understood immediately.

There is no doubt that, if the numbers of parents benefiting from antenatal education is to be increased, innovative schemes are required; such schemes may be demanding on educators' time and resources, but the spin-off could be considerable in reducing postnatal unhappiness and depression, and in improving the quality of parenting.

KEY POINTS

- **Underprivileged women, although at increased risk of having a premature or poorly baby, do not usually attend antenatal classes.**

- **Childbirth education aims not only to help every parent prepare for birth and parenting, but also to provide a positive experience of education which will encourage parents to create a learning environment in their own homes.**

- **Before they can deliver a sensitive and useful service to any parent, childbirth educators need to explore and resolve their own prejudices.**

- **Cultural sensitivity is most easily and fully achieved when childbirth educators are recruited from the ethnic group itself.**

- **The self-esteem of women and couples with physical, mental, psychological or social difficulties is enhanced when childbirth educators help them become more confident in their abilities to do what 'normal' women/couples do.**

- **The major challenge facing childbirth education today is to be equally accessible to every parent.**

- **Parents with particular needs may benefit from receiving childbirth education within a peer group, but including them in mainstream antenatal classes integrates them into 'normal' parental life.**

REFERENCES

Avery P and McKenzie I (1987) Expanding the scope of childbirth education to meet the needs of hospitalized, high-risk clients. *Journal of Obstetric, Gynaecological and Neonatal Nursing* **November/December**: 418–420.

Campion MJ (1990) *The Baby Challenge: A Handbook on Pregnancy for Women with a Physical Disability*. London: Tavistock Routledge.

Carty E and Conine T (1993) The childbearing and parenting program for women with disabilities/chronic illness. In *Midwives: Hear the Heartbeat of the Future. Proceedings of the International Confederation of Midwives 23rd International Congress*, 9–14 May 1993, Vol. 1, pp 373–374. Vancouver: ICM.

Chadwick J (1994) Perinatal mortality and antenatal care. *Modern Midwife* **4**(9): 18.

Dixon K (1996) Practical tips for supporting pregnant women with learning disabilities (1). *Disability, Pregnancy and Parenthood International* Issue No. 15, October 1996.

Edwards J (1995) Provision of antenatal classes for black and ethnic minority women in Preston. *MIDIRS Midwifery Digest* **5**(4): 412–413.

Hancock A (1994) How effective is antenatal education? *Modern Midwife* **4**(5): 13.

Hartman A and Laird J (1990) Family treatment after adoption – common themes. In Brodzinsky DM and Schechter MD (eds) *The Psychology of Adoption*. Oxford: Oxford University Press.

Hay DA, Gleeson C and Davies C (1990) What information should the multiple births family receive before, during and after birth? *Acta Geneticae Medicae Gemellologiae* **39**: 259–269.

Hudson F and Ineichen B (1994) *Taking it Lying Down: Sexuality and Teenage Motherhood*. London: Macmillan Education.

Jeffers D (1992) Outreach childbirth education classes for low income families: a strategy for program development. *International Journal of Childbirth Education* **7**(3): 17–18.

Mander R (1994) *Loss and Bereavement in Childbearing*. Oxford: Blackwell Scientific Publications.

McEwan Carty E, Conine T and Hall L (1990) Comprehensive health promotion for the pregnant woman who is disabled. *Journal of Nurse-Midwifery* **35**(3): 134–136.

McGrail A (1996) *Becoming a Family*. London: National Childbirth Trust in collaboration with HMSO.

Meikle S, Orleans M, Leff M, Shain R and Gibbs R (1995) Women's reasons for not seeking prenatal care: racial and ethnic factors. *Birth* **22**(2): 81–86.

Montgomery K (1991) Taking outreach a giant step further. *International Journal of Childbirth Education* **10**: 10–11.

Newton Verrier N (1994) *The Primal Wound: Understanding the Adopted Child*. Baltimore: Gateway Press.

Nolan, M (1996) Teenage pregnancy: meeting the need – the Blenheim/Harding Trust. *Modern Midwife* November 1996: 22–24.

Pattberg R (1997) Lesbian parents. *International Journal of Childbirth Education* **12**(2): 20.

Pugh G, De'Ath E and Smith C (1994) *Confident Parents, Confident Children: Policy and Practice in Parent Education and Support*. London: National Children's Bureau.

Redman S, Oak S, Booth P, Jensen J and Saxton A (1991) Evaluation of an antenatal education programme: characteristics of attenders, changes in knowledge and satisfaction of participants. *Australian and New Zealand Journal of Obstetrics and Gynaecology* **31**(4): 310–316.

Sturrock WA and Johnson J (1990) The relationship between childbirth education classes and obstetric outcomes. *Birth* **17**(2): 82–85.

Thorpe K, Golding J, MacGillivray I et al (1991) Comparison of prevalence of depression in mothers of twins and mothers of singletons. *British Medical Journal* **302**: 875–878.

Walker J and Pollard E (1995) Parent education for Asian mothers. *Modern Midwife* **5**(9): 22–23.

Young D (1990) How can we 'enrich' prenatal care? *Birth* **17**(1): 12–13.

Challenging Teaching Situations 11

PROVIDING ANTENATAL EDUCATION TO VERY LARGE GROUPS

It is difficult to justify delivering antenatal education to groups consisting of very large numbers of people. Whilst it may be feasible to transmit information to such groups in lecture format, it is not possible to respond to individual learning needs in any way that permits the name of 'education' to be applied to the situation. None the less, the reality of contemporary antenatal education is such that limited resources often force educators into a position where they are obliged to hand out information in just such an impersonal fashion. It would be useful to research what exactly parents gain from attending the 'pain relief lecture' or the 'breastfeeding lecture', but it is reasonable to presume that the level of such lectures is pitched too high for some, too low for others, and that they fail to assist parents in applying information to their personal situations. Whilst questions from the floor may be invited, it is a commonly observed phenomenon that only people with great confidence or who are used to speaking in public situations avail themselves of such opportunities. These are not the people who have difficulty accessing information.

Childbirth educators need to have a political agenda that includes raising the status of antenatal education so that managers do not consider it appropriate or acceptable to provide classes for large groups of people whose individual differences cannot thereby be catered for. The influence that antenatal education can have on people at a time when they are unusually open to looking at themselves and their lives is reduced if educators are unable to engage in a personal dialogue. Quine and colleagues' analysis of failures of communication between health carers and their clients is particularly pertinent when considered in the light of antenatal education offered to huge numbers of parents:

> Patients' failure to understand stems from three interrelated problems: the material presented to them is often too difficult to understand; patients sometimes do not understand basic physiology or anatomy and often lack

elementary medical knowledge about their own bodies; patients often have active misconceptions that are so incorrect as to interfere with proper comprehension. (Quine et al, 1993, p 112)

Whilst information is important, it is insufficient without the opportunity to check that it has been understood and applied. However, given that limited resources and the lack of status of antenatal education are likely to mean that educators will continue to find themselves working with large groups of parents and their supporters, it is necessary to consider how learning can be facilitated in such circumstances. Every large group is made up of individuals, and the individuality of parents needs to be acknowledged and their connection with other parents fostered. There are a number of techniques for the childbirth educator to employ:

1. At the beginning of the session, invite each person present to introduce him or herself to someone else in the group. Introductions are easier if the educator suggests some topics for conversation such as when the baby is due, intended place of birth, how the pregnancy has been so far, etc.

2. At the end of each section of the talk, invite people to discuss with the person in front or behind or next to them how they feel about what has been said.

3. Keep the content of the talk as simple as possible, aiming to transmit only the most important facts.

4. Use a variety of teaching aids to assist understanding – pictures, overheads, dolls, models of the pelvis, the educator's own body . . .

5. If the talk is a long one, and certainly if it is more than 1 hour in length, invite people to stand at some point and do a simple shake and stretch exercise to revive their concentration.

6. At the end of the talk, invite people to group into fours or sixes and identify any questions they want to put. Take one question from each group in turn.

7. As people are leaving, be available to answer any outstanding questions that parents may prefer to ask on a one-to-one basis.

Penny Simkin, a well known American childbirth educator, advocates the use of 'class assistants' when teaching large groups (Simkin, 1984). These may be student teachers or parents who have recently had their babies. The assistants welcome people as they arrive for the session and help facilitate small group work. Simkin invites class attenders to telephone her after the session if they have material they want to discuss further. She maintains that it *is* possible to provide a satisfactory learning experience for large groups (by which she means up to 30 people):

Teaching large groups means changing one's teaching style, using good assistants, facilitating formation of subgroups of (parents) with similar interests, creating a warm, open atmosphere which encourages people to share feelings and concerns, and placing the burden on the (parents) to help make sure they get their needs met. (Simkin, 1984, p 177)

Providing Antenatal Education to Very Small Groups

Educators may sometimes find themselves facilitating sessions for a very few parents and their supporters. This is not as easy as it sounds. The intimacy of a small group puts everyone on the spot in a way which the relative anonymity of a larger group avoids. On the other hand, the educator has the chance to get to know her group well and so is able to devise learning experiences that are very specific to people's needs. An immense amount of learning can be achieved in a fairly short period of time. Information sharing and discussion can be clearly focused on what it is that each person wants to know or talk about. Everybody in the group can have the chance to practise babycare skills; everybody can handle the pelvis and put the doll through it.

Parents who are part of a very small group do not have the same scope as members of a larger one to choose the people whom they would like to incorporate into their support network – there is no reason why two couples who are the only members of their antenatal class should necessarily get on. It is therefore important for the educator working with a small group to help parents explore their support options, and to ensure they know about other groups they can join after the birth of their babies.

Perhaps the greatest challenge for the educator working with a very small group is to provide non-threatening opportunities for practising self-help skills for labour. People are likely to be very self-conscious when trying out different positions, practising massage and breathing through imaginary contractions if they feel closely observed by other group members and the educator herself. It is, however, vital to encourage such practice in classes and a number of strategies may be employed to help maximize learning value and minimize awkwardness:

1. The educator can participate in the practical work herself.

2. She needs to give clear instructions to group members so that everyone is quite sure what he or she is being invited to do.

3. If the room is large enough, each mother and her supporter can be encouraged to choose a private corner where the two can work with their backs to other people in the room.

4. Dimming the lights helps people feel more private and less conscious of one another.

5. The educator needs to talk the group members through the work they are doing and offer constructive and reassuring feedback.

Providing Antenatal Education to Groups that Include Only First-time Parents

With a group consisting entirely of parents expecting their first babies, the educator may feel relieved that she can 'begin at the beginning' and work through the course content without the need to respond to and integrate the possibly complicated and distressing experiences of people who have previously given birth and cared for newborn babies. This assumption is, of course, almost bound to be erroneous. None of the first-time parents will really be a clean slate as far as antenatal education is concerned. Amongst the group, there will inevitably be some women who have had miscarriages, some people whose pregnancy is the result of an assisted conception, some parents who have relatives or friends who have burdened them with undigested accounts of their own labours, perhaps one or two women who have previously had a late abortion. A 'round robin' exercise at the beginning of the first or second class with each group member being asked to complete the sentence 'Labour is . . .' may well elicit responses indicative of a huge range of experiences which people in the group have already gone through.

The educator can adopt various strategies to help parents expecting their first babies reflect on what they already know about labour, birth and early parenting. She can invite group members to discuss the old wives' tales they have been told and to share the experiences they have already had, at first or second hand, in relation to childbearing.

BOX 11.1 WHAT DO YOU ALREADY KNOW ABOUT LABOUR AND BIRTH?

Aim

> to raise group members' awareness of their own prejudices about labour and birth

Learning outcome

> group members will be able to identify the influences on their ideas about labour and birth

In small groups, invite parents and supporters to construct a list of all the positive things they have heard about labour, and all the negative things.

Ask for feedback into the whole group. Useful questions to put may be:

- **Why is it that labour is so often portrayed on television as a horrendous experience? (Clement, 1997)**

- **How does what you have heard about labour make you feel now that it is your turn?**

- **How do you cope with other people's negative accounts of labour?**

- **What do you think would have helped some of the people you know who had very unpleasant labours?**

Such an exercise will enable the educator to correct any wrong information that group members hold, to identify particular areas of concern and to begin to help parents identify their own ways of coping with labour.

Educators can broaden the understanding of first-time parents by providing opportunities for them to hear, in a structured learning environment rather than casually, accounts of the labours and early parenting experiences of other people. Birth reports (Kitzinger, 1971; Gaskin, 1990; Limburg and Smulders, 1992) can be read out during class to give a flavour of the huge amount of variation possible even within normal labour. Parents who have recently given birth can be invited to the class with their babies to share their experiences. Such a visit is an essential component of antenatal education for groups composed entirely of primiparous women and their supporters. The presence of a baby not only helps make their own babies real to women who have not yet borne a child and to their partners, but also acts as a stimulant for the many questions that first-time parents need answered about babycare and postnatal life.

The educator needs to be sure that the visiting parents have had an opportunity before the class to debrief their experiences (see Chapter 5).

WORKING WITH CHALLENGING PEOPLE IN ANTENATAL CLASSES

Providing antenatal education for small groups sometimes means that childbirth educators must confront problems posed by group members whose efforts to grapple with their fears and uncertainties about the transition to parenthood make it difficult for others to learn in peace. No matter how experienced the educator, she is likely to find certain types of behaviour and certain people difficult to handle. People who:

- dominate every discussion
- say nothing
- show by their verbal and non-verbal behaviour that they are extremely anxious
- clearly do not want to be at the class
- do not want to participate in practical work
- set themselves up as the class jokers
- undermine everything the educator says
- are extremely knowledgeable and/or are childbirth professionals

constitute an enormous part of the challenge of delivering high-quality antenatal education in groups. These are the people who stretch an educator's skills to their limit and enable her to challenge herself and her teaching to the ultimate benefit of both.

MEETING THE NEEDS OF VERY TALKATIVE GROUP MEMBERS

The childbirth educator needs to try to understand why people who challenge at antenatal classes behave as they do. It may be that the person who talks too much is the most anxious person in the group. Anxiety may be the result of uncertainty about the norms of an antenatal class – 'like entering a women's masonic lodge' was how one man described going to antenatal classes (Schott, 1996) – or it may be generated by fear of childbirth or ambivalence about impending parenthood. Overly talkative people may not be used to being listened to and therefore do not listen. The educator has to avoid labelling such group members as 'difficult' and marginalizing them, but rather she has to help them learn. Teaching strategies to encourage a talkative person to listen might include:

1. identifying her particular area of concern and making this a topic for small group work, or taking the opportunity during a break to speak to her about her particular worries

2. using small group work and placing the talkative person with other articulate and assertive people who are likely to insist on having their say

3. using small group work and making it a ground rule that every person in the group must have a couple of minutes to express his or her opinion or thoughts

4. inviting feedback after small group work from spokespersons who do not include the talkative class member

5. placing the teaching doll in the middle of the room when a discussion is in progress and allowing only the person holding the baby to speak

6. using people's names to invite them to contribute to the discussion

7. inviting each member of the group to say something in turn (a 'round robin')

8. if absolutely necessary, challenging a group member directly: 'You've put your point of view, Peter; now Leroy wants to say something.'

Very often, other group members will be successful in controlling the behaviour of one of their number who is impeding learning. Non-verbal communication such as raised eyebrows, crossed arms, averted eyes, sighs and disinterested expressions may be correctly interpreted by the obtrusive member who will then modify his or her behaviour accordingly. The educator's responsibility, however, is to try to meet the learning needs of every member of the group and this means being available to each person no matter how difficult she finds his or her attitudes or behaviour to be. By creating a welcoming atmosphere in the class, showing that she has a sincere interest in everyone's well-being, demonstrating her listening skills and valuing what each group member has to say, the educator may succeed in reassuring overly talkative parents or supporters that they do not need to fight for acceptance within the group and that their needs will be granted equal status with everyone else's.

MEETING THE NEEDS OF VERY QUIET GROUP MEMBERS

It can be even more difficult for educators to assess the learning needs of class members who say nothing at all than those of very talkative individuals. Some people are naturally reticent, but none the less listen carefully to what is being said, apply it silently to their own situation and are, judging from their body language, completely engaged with the subject under discussion. They are different from those who are silent because they are terrified or ambivalent about pregnancy, childbirth, parenting and/or antenatal classes.

Particularly anxious women are often those who have what psychotherapists describe as 'overvalued' pregnancies. These are women whose pregnancy follows prolonged efforts to have a baby, or who are having a first baby in their late thirties or forties, or who have experienced recurrent miscarriages or an ectopic pregnancy, or a stillbirth, or who have given birth to a baby with a disability. Such women may find it impossible to relax and enjoy their pregnancy even when it is well established and the first critical months are over:

> Many such women experience the need to 'monitor' the pregnancy continuously as if their vigil keeps the baby in existence and even a fleeting loss of concentration will result in it vanishing . . . For these women, unassisted waiting is intolerable and they will often present with hyperchondriacal anxieties which are a cry for psychological help.
> (Raphael-Leff, 1993, p 95)

There may be great anxiety amongst pregnant class members for other reasons. Women who are survivors of abuse may dread the public nature of contemporary childbirth – being exposed to the eyes of strangers and subjected to intimate examinations which revive memories of abuse and hurt (Parratt, 1994). Women with a history of psychiatric illness may find their mental health fragile when faced with even the ordinary stresses of pregnancy. Women who are under pressure for religious, cultural or familial reasons to have a male baby (less commonly, a female) are also likely to be particularly anxious.

Well facilitated groups are generally very sensitive to the needs of their individual members. Overly anxious parents or supporters are likely to find they are well cared for if given the chance to get to know and confide in other members of the class. The childbirth educator may need to set time aside to offer an anxious person a listening ear so that some of her fears are unloaded during class breaks or over the telephone, leaving more space for other members of the group during classes. With the permission of the individual, the educator may deem it appropriate to consult with medical or midwifery colleagues if she suspects that an underlying physical or psychiatric illness is responsible for excessive anxiety.

Class members who are naturally quiet and those who are frightened and afraid to communicate their fears are likely to be helped by working in small groups. Whilst speaking out in a group of 16 would be impossible for them, contributing to a discussion amongst four people may be quite manageable. If a class contains many people who are unwilling to contribute in the large group, small group work must be the backbone of the antenatal course. The educator can boost the self-esteem of quiet people by taking note of what they say in their small groups and, if the material is not confidential, referring to their comments in the whole group. People are generally pleased to find their ideas taken up by the group leader and may be encouraged to speak more freely afterwards.

MEETING THE NEEDS OF PEOPLE WHO ARE RELUCTANT TO BE AT CLASSES

For the most part, people who come to antenatal classes have chosen to attend and are keen to learn. Sometimes, a father may have been persuaded to attend against his will, and, occasionally, the situation is the reverse one where the person who is to be the labour supporter feels the need for antenatal education and support but the pregnant woman does not. People who do not want to be at classes may (a) decide to make the best of a bad situation and see whether there is anything to be gained from it or (b) refuse to participate in any discussion or activity or be deliberately disruptive. Those in the first category are easily won over if the classes are dynamic, well structured and cater for the needs and interests of every group member. People in the second may be helped to enjoy the learning opportunities provided if the educator can encourage them by using some of the strategies already identified in this chapter to modify their behaviour. Class attenders whose behaviour is relentlessly disruptive, however, and which jeopardizes the learning of other group members may need to be challenged. People have the right *not* to attend antenatal classes and it is sometimes appropriate for the educator to ask whether a particular individual wants to make the choice not to attend again. This could have implications for the person with whom he or she is coming to classes and the educator may have the difficult task of talking to both in order to identify how the needs and preferences of each can best be met.

Reluctant attenders may cover their discomfiture and resentment at being forced to do something they don't want to do by making a joke of everything that is said, and taking any opportunity to sidetrack discussions. Antenatal education should be challenging and some-times engage class members in topics that are frightening; however, there is a natural tendency on the part of any group to turn away from heavy topics and the class joker may be used as a means of avoiding difficult issues. Whilst the atmosphere in classes may feel very light-hearted as a consequence, it is almost certain that the educator will be attacked on the clients' evaluation forms for her failure to help the group accomplish any useful work. If the group itself is not strong enough to control the joker, the educator must help. She may need to step in to put discussions back on track after interruptions have occurred and employ strategies similar to those for coping with talkative class members in order to ensure that the class agenda is not thwarted. In the last resort, she may have to tackle the disruptive person on his own, point out that he is disrupting the group and ask for his cooperation. This requires a lot of courage and the educator should seek the support of colleagues in planning for and debriefing such a confrontation.

MEETING THE NEEDS OF PEOPLE WHO ARE EXTREMELY KNOWLEDGEABLE

Many childbirth educators dread the presence of health professionals in their groups, fearing that they may have come only to criticize the content of the course, to undermine the educator or to demonstrate how well informed they themselves are. Considered rationally, this is highly unlikely to be the case. Health professionals, no matter how experienced and even if they are maternity care specialists, will be just as vulnerable and just as anxious as any other parent (if not more so) when they become pregnant. Often, because their carers expect them to know about pregnancy and labour and how to look after babies, they receive far less information and support than 'ordinary' parents. What they may long for, above all else, is to be treated simply as a pregnant mother or father, allowed to express their fears, ask their questions and become part of a support group of people in similar circumstances.

Often, health professionals are happy not to give any indication that they have specialist knowledge and thoroughly enjoy being accepted on equal terms by other group members. Some educators make it their principle never to provide an opportunity for class members to say what job they do. This avoids the almost inevitable feeling on the part of some group members that their job (and therefore their contributions to classes) is inferior to somebody else's, and the risk that parents will expect the group members who are health professionals to run the group and be the key people in every discussion and activity. If the educator herself does not know what parents and their supporters do for a living, she may well be more clear-sighted in understanding the particular needs that have brought them to classes.

Occasionally, a health professional who is attending classes wants to share his or her expertise and this can be welcomed by the educator as a useful opportunity for group members to broaden their knowledge and gain insight into the problems that health carers face in their work. However, when information or opinions are offered too frequently or simply, it would seem, for the sake of 'showing off', the educator needs to try to understand what is at the root of that person's desire to demonstrate that he or she is more knowledgeable than everyone else. Perhaps the reason is insecurity; the knowledgeable person attempts to control the emotions and fears that pregnancy and the anticipation of labour generate by constant self-reassurance that he or she is more than sufficiently knowledgeable to cope with the situation.

While health professionals may not need to learn about the anatomy and physiology of birth, they may well need to explore their emotions in relation to becoming a parent or being a labour supporter. Small group work that centres on feelings and coping strategies rather than sharing factual information may encourage people with medical expertise to address the areas that are important for them.

SUMMARY

The challenges and rewards of antenatal education arise from the variety of teaching situations in which the educator may find herself. No matter whether the group with which she is working is very large or very small, consists only of parents expecting their first babies or includes multiparous parents as well, is composed entirely of health professionals or entirely of people who know nothing about how babies are born, the principles of working with the clients' agenda, building on the knowledge and skills people already have, and providing a broad range of learning opportunities, always hold good. Group members who do not conform to the unwritten etiquette of antenatal classes challenge the educator to explore why their behaviour is different and to find ways in which they can be helped to learn or, in the last resort, prevented from hindering the learning of others. Educating, like learning, is a dynamic process and the presence of non-typical people in an antenatal group is a spur to the educator's personal and professional development.

KEY POINTS

1. **Every first-time parent comes to classes with some knowledge, accurate or otherwise, and some experience, at first or second hand, of childbirth and parenting.**

2. **Very anxious group members are likely to find they are well cared for by other people in the group if the educator creates a safe environment in her classes.**

3. **Group members who challenge may simply be expressing their fears and uncertainties about the transition to parenthood.**

REFERENCES

Clement S (1997) Childbirth on Television. *British Journal of Midwifery* **5**(1): 37–40.

Gaskin IM (1990) *Spiritual Midwifery*. Summertown, Tennessee: The Book Publishing Company.

Kitzinger S (1971) *Giving Birth: The Parents' Emotions in Childbirth*. London: Gollancz.

Limburg A and Smulders B (1992) *Women Giving Birth*. Berkeley, California: Celestial Arts Publishing.

Parratt J (1994) The experience of childbirth for survivors of incest. *Midwifery* **10**: 26–39.

Quine L, Rutter DR and Gowen S (1993) Women's satisfaction with the quality of the birth experience: a prospective study of social and psychological predictors. *Journal of Reproductive and Infant Psychology* **11**: 107–113.

Raphael-Leff J (1993) *Psychological Processes of Childbearing*. London: Chapman and Hall.

Schott J (1996) Speaking at 'Changing Childbirth, Challenging Antenatal Education', National Childbirth Trust Conference, 23 November 1996, Bournemouth, UK.

Simkin P (1984) Effective childbirth education: are small classes the only way? *Birth* **11**(3): 176–177.

12 Evaluating Teaching

In the beginning, most people, whether they are childbirth educators or educators in any other subject, are concerned mainly with the content of their classes and whether they manage to cover the essential material in the time available. They are anxious that they may be asked questions that they cannot answer or find themselves attempting to explain things to their students that they are not quite clear about themselves. It is characteristic of adult education classes that there is nearly always somebody amongst the learners who has more technical knowledge than the educator herself, or who has more immediate experience of the subject under discussion. This is not a problem – the knowledge held by the clients, and their previous experiences, are a treasure chest which the educator can dip into at regular intervals and share with the rest of the group. Much of the pleasure of learning as far as clients are concerned is to discover that they already have much of the information they need.

Once concern about the content of classes becomes less pressing, the educator is in a position to start observing herself and her clients more closely.

You can make judgments about how you are working with individual students, how you taught a particular session, and about your work and achievement for a whole course.
(Daines et al, 1994, p 86)

The ability to stand back and to see herself and listen to herself as others are seeing her and listening to her is an essential part of the process of evaluation without which no educator improves her skills.

Evaluation takes place in three stages:

1. The educator observes her own teaching and the responses of her clients.

2. She analyses her observations.

3. She devises strategies to enable her to meet the needs of her clients more effectively on the next occasion when she teaches.

Evaluation starts, as does teaching itself, with aims and learning outcomes. Unless the educator has defined for herself what it is she hopes her clients will gain from her antenatal classes, both in global terms, and in precise measurable terms, she is in no position to evaluate whether she has been effective as a childbirth educator and whether parents have benefited from spending their time with her.

AIMS

Aims are expressed in terms that do not lend themselves to precise measurement (see Chapter 2). They encompass the educator's philosophy of antenatal education and summarize the motivating forces that drive her to try to make her classes as good as possible. They demonstrate that she *believes* in the value of preparation for birth and parenting and is totally committed to it. She can perhaps never say, with certainty, that she has achieved her aims, because how can she know whether:

- she has inspired the parents in her classes with confidence in women's ability to give birth?

- she has boosted their confidence that they are the best people to make decisions about their children?

- she has promoted postnatal mental health?

- she has enabled parents to participate more fully in their own care?

None the less, aims remain the cornerstone on which the childbirth educator builds her classes. Evidence as to whether or not she has achieved them cannot be provided in statistical terms, but may be gleaned in other ways which are discussed in this chapter.

LEARNING OUTCOMES

When asked to evaluate a class, many educators will respond in such terms as:

'I think it went really well.'

'Everyone had a laugh.'

'It was good fun.'

'The group just didn't gel.'

These are 'gut' reactions and are quite permissible. Every educator is allowed to have feelings about her classes, and to use her instinct to assess whether or not she enabled people to learn. She may 'know' in her heart that a particular class was not successful and that her clients were bored and learnt very little even if she cannot quite define in her head why her teaching approaches were not effective. The importance and legitimacy of gut reactions should never be denied. However, they cannot be the sole means by which the educator evaluates her effectiveness. She needs to seek more concrete evidence as to whether her classes provided useful learning experiences for the people attending them. She has to ask herself what she means by a class that 'went really well' and whether it went really well for her (in that she covered the material she had set out to cover) or for the parents and their supporters (in that they were enabled to learn things which *they* considered to be useful).

Learning outcomes (see Chapter 2) enable the educator to assess whether the learning she and her clients hoped would be achieved actually was achieved. They enable her to ask herself, for example, whether class members did acquire some babycare and self-help skills for labour, whether parents and their supporters did expand and consolidate the information they had on a particular topic, and whether clients were able to identify hopes, feelings and expectations in relation to birth and early parenting. Learning outcomes are dependent on the variety of learning experiences that the educator provides during her class. If outcomes are not achieved, the educator needs to ask herself whether this was because parents wanted to do different work from what she had planned, or whether it was because she lacked the confidence to provide a particular learning opportunity, or whether it was because she allowed a discussion to outlast its usefulness, so leaving no time for another important learning activity. Learning outcomes should be assessed after each class to see whether they have been achieved, and to enable any that have been missed to be achieved in future classes.

OBSERVING CLIENTS

Everything class members say or do provides the childbirth educator with evidence about whether she is helping them to learn or not. The more skilled an observer of her own clients she is, the more able she will be to facilitate useful learning opportunities.

People's body language is a primary source of information about their involvement in the class. The mother who is constantly shifting in her seat, trying to ease her back, rubbing her bump, or crossing and uncrossing her legs is telling the educator, without words, that she is uncomfortable, that she has backache, that her baby is pressing on a nerve and that she needs to move. It is a very simple fact, but one that is frequently overlooked by childbirth educators, that pregnant women (or indeed, any person in whatever condition) cannot learn unless they are physically comfortable. In the situation described above, the childbirth educator needs to recognize the woman's discomfort and provide an opportunity for everyone to move either by doing some physical skills work or by breaking the large group into smaller groups or by offering a coffee break. The evidence is clear, even if unspoken, that this woman is not learning anything from the class because she is being distracted by the physical demands of her pregnant body.

Similarly, people who are yawning, reading the posters on the classroom wall or gazing into space are not learning. The father (or mother or labour supporter) who is sitting so that he is half turned away from the childbirth educator may be making a different statement. He may feel frightened by the subject the group is discussing, uncomfortable with topics that seem to him very intimate, or uncertain about his own role in the class. If the childbirth educator is aware of his body language, she may be able to think of ways of helping him feel more relaxed in order to improve his learning experience.

Practical skills work offers the educator a wealth of information about how couples are feeling about their pregnancy and the impending birth, and about how relaxed they are with their own bodies. In one of her own classes, the author observed how seven of the eight couples in her group responded with alacrity to a suggestion that the woman might stand and lean on her partner during a contraction, while the eighth (a doctor and senior nurse) found it too embarrassing to put their arms round each other in public and practise coping with a contraction. This is the kind of evidence that requires the educator to 'think on her feet' and adapt her teaching approaches almost from minute to minute in order to ensure that every parent finds her class an individually tailored and effective learning experience. In the case mentioned above, the author suggested that the woman might lean against the wall whilst her partner massaged her lower back. This enabled the couple to turn away from the rest of the group and to create a private space of their own.

Observation of the group also includes noting who is contributing to discussion and who is not, whether certain people are preventing others from joining in and whether there are people who never say anything. The educator needs to decide whether quiet people are quiet because they are intimidated or because they choose to be. Not everyone wants to hold centre stage; some people keep their ideas to themselves, but are not necessarily learning less than more talkative members of the group. A mother who is leaning forward in her seat, making eye contact with the person who is speaking, responding to what is being said with nods and 'mmm's, is clearly engaged with the topic in hand, even if she is not contributing directly to the discussion.

Listening to the kind of questions being asked gives the educator further clues as to the quality of the learning taking place within the group. Questions that ask for facts reflect a desire on the part of the questioner to increase his or her confidence through knowledge. However, antenatal classes where people ask only for facts and never speculate may be failing to confront the broader emotional and philosophical issues to do with making health choices. Open-ended questions indicate a desire to explore feelings, to project into unfamiliar situations and to empathize with the experience of others; for example:

'How is my boss going to feel if I'm expressing milk in the coffee break?!'

'Is it realistic to expect the midwife to go along with our ideas if she doesn't agree with them?'

In a well balanced class, group members should be asking both open-ended and closed questions.

The childbirth educator can assess her relationship with the group – whether she is acting as a facilitator or is seen as the leader with all the answers – by noting whether people tend to address their comments to her, or whether they talk to each other without feeling the need always to bounce their ideas off her first. It is helpful to draw a diagram of the interactions that are occurring (Figure 12.1).

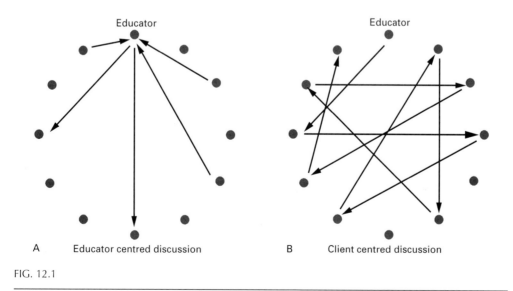

| A | Educator centred discussion | B | Client centred discussion |

FIG. 12.1

If the first situation applies, the educator may want to consider whether she is effectively promoting self-reliance amongst the parents in her class, or whether she is setting herself up as a guru and encouraging parents to seek the answers to every question from a professional source. The second diagram is more likely to represent a group where parents are sharing information with each other, problem-solving together and learning to support each other without becoming over-reliant on a professional care-giver.

Discussion should always be a feature of antenatal classes, but the fact that people are talking to each other either in small groups or in the whole group does not, in itself, indicate that useful learning is taking place. While it is legitimate and desirable for there to be a certain amount of banter in classes and for people to exchange their news, this needs to be balanced by opportunities to explore in depth the topics that are central to antenatal education. Evaluating the success of classes therefore involves asking whether discussion enabled people to acknowledge their feelings or whether it remained superficial and 'safe', skirting round emotive issues. Body language offers clues as to how deeply people are engaged in what they are talking about: frowns of concentration, questioning looks, nods of agreement, shakes of the head, hand gestures – all of these suggest that people are really hearing what is being said and are relating it to their own experience.

The childbirth educator needs to evaluate how much information people have gained during the course. She may do this by asking the group to feed back to her the important points about, for example, the onset of labour. She will also be able to tell how much people have retained by noting whether the questions they ask at one class are derived from information acquired at an earlier one, whether they are able to make connections between topics, and whether practical work reveals that they are bringing together all the skills they have learnt to date.

OVERALL IMPRESSION

After dissecting her class in this way, it is important for the educator to consider its overall impact and 'feel'. She can substantiate her gut reactions by answering such questions as:

1   What was the atmosphere like during this class? Were the parents:

interested	bored	active
chatty	silent	friendly
hostile	confused	restless
anxious	involved	

2   What was the pace of the class like? Was it:

slow	tedious	lively
fast	frantic	stimulating
repetitious		

Looking at the balance of teaching approaches used during the class also provides the educator with evidence about the quality of the overall learning experience, bearing in mind that people have different learning styles and that everyone benefits from a variety of learning opportunities:

3   Teaching techniques used were:

lecture	discussion	demonstration
small group work	practical skills work	role play
work in couples	brainstorming	

The educator should also challenge herself about her standards of preparation:

4   How well prepared was I for this class?

not at all	insufficiently	adequately
very well	outstandingly	

5   What visual aids did I use?

- Did I display/handle them in such a way that everybody could see?
- Did they help people to understand the topic better?
- Could they have been used more effectively? How?

6   Was the environment of the class comfortable with regard to:

- lighting
- heating
- seating arrangements
- space for practical skills work
- cleanliness
- toilet facilities
- refreshments?

ASKING CLIENTS FOR FEEDBACK

Detailed and honest observation of classes by the educator herself provides her with excellent feedback regarding effectiveness. There are two other important ways of obtaining feedback. The first of these is to ask clients for their opinion.

The majority of today's adults lead extremely busy lives; they value their time and will not waste it attending classes they find boring or which do not help them to learn about the things they are concerned about. People often vote with their feet if they are dissatisfied with their antenatal classes, and simply fail to turn up. It is, of course, extremely disheartening for an educator to find the number of her clients dwindling from week to week. However, if she can put her feelings of hurt to one side, she can ask herself whether there is some external reason for the poor uptake (attendance at the best antenatal classes is sporadic during bank holiday weekends!) or whether parents are telling her that her classes are not meeting their needs. If the drift away from classes appears to be related to their content and presentation, the educator needs to seek support in order to explore why they are not being perceived as useful by parents.

The easiest way to obtain feedback from clients (although not necessarily the most effective because people do not always give a straight answer to a straight question) is to ask at the end of each class whether group members have enjoyed it:

- Was today's class useful?

- What did you enjoy doing most?

- What didn't you enjoy?

- Have you any worries about what we have done today?

It is an excellent idea to provide an opportunity half-way through the antenatal course for people to say whether they are satisfied with the classes and to suggest any changes they would like to make. Group members' views can be sought either verbally or by asking them to complete a short questionnaire. The childbirth educator can then adapt her teaching approaches to tailor them more closely to the group's learning needs for the second half of the course.

Groups whose members trust and respect their educator will probably be prepared to offer an honest verbal evaluation of classes. However, people often find it hard to voice their criticisms, and verbal feedback may need to be supplemented with written. It is important to understand how to construct a feedback form to ensure that it generates information that will help the educator consider how to improve her teaching. Many childbirth educators hand out evaluation forms at the end of their courses, but find that they yield little information of service to them. These are some of the important points to bear in mind:

1. Everyone hates filling in long questionnaires. If possible, the questionnaire should be kept to one side of an A4 sheet.

2. Two questions should not be rolled into one, for example:

- Were the visits of the breastfeeding counsellor and the new parents helpful?

(This question is difficult to respond to if people enjoyed one visit but not the other.)

3. A mix of closed and open-ended questions is desirable. An evaluation form composed entirely of closed questions does not give people the chance to express a range of feelings. On the other hand, evaluation forms that ask only open-ended questions take a long time to complete. Not everyone will be prepared to put in the necessary effort.

4. It is useful to ask a colleague to read through the evaluation form before it is distributed to see whether she understands all the questions.

5. When to hand out evaluation forms and how to collect them in again are critical issues. The educator can set aside 10 minutes during the final class for people to complete the forms and hand them back to her. This ensures a 100% return rate. If parents are given evaluation forms to complete after their babies are born so that they can reflect on the usefulness of their classes in the light of the experiences they have had, they can be asked to leave the forms on the postnatal ward or hand them to their community midwife. If forms are given to clients to take away and send back by post, very few are likely to be returned.

6. Every person attending the antenatal course should fill in an evaluation form; one form per couple will not tell the educator whether her classes are meeting the needs of the women *and* the men/labour supporters in her group.

The evaluation form needs itself to be evaluated; if clients are giving useful feedback to the childbirth educator so that she can work on improving her teaching, it is serving its purpose. If, however, feedback is thin, the evaluation form needs redesigning. It is worthwhile experimenting with different kinds of evaluation forms to see which format is best. (See Box 12.1)

BOX 12.1 EVALUATION FORM

Please complete and return to ....

1. During these antenatal classes, I have learned: (please circle)

   a great deal   quite a lot   enough   a little   nothing

2. As a whole, the classes have been: (please circle)

   excellent   very good   good   adequate   poor

3. I would like: (please tick those that apply)

   less lecture ☐   less practical ☐   less group discussion ☐

   more lecture ☐   more practical ☐   more group discussion ☐

   the balance of methods is about right ☐

4. What I found most helpful about the classes was:

5. What I liked least about the classes was:

6. In future courses, I would suggest:

7. Further comments:

BOX 12.2 EVALUATION FORM

Please complete and return to . . . . before the end of the class.

1. How useful were the antenatal classes in terms of: (please tick one number for each item)

	Extremely useful				Useless
Learning about what happens in labour	1	2	3	4	5
Practising self-help skills for labour	1	2	3	4	5
Gaining confidence about communicating with health professionals	1	2	3	4	5
Learning about caesarean section	1	2	3	4	5
Learning about the drugs used for pain relief in labour	1	2	3	4	5
Learning about breastfeeding	1	2	3	4	5
Discussing life changes after the birth of my baby	1	2	3	4	5
Practising babycare skills	1	2	3	4	5
Finding out about sex and contraception after the birth of my baby	1	2	3	4	5
Getting to know other people expecting babies	1	2	3	4	5
Exchanging ideas with other people	1	2	3	4	5

2. Are there any topics that you consider should have been included and weren't?

3. Are there any further comments you would like to make?

It is always daunting to sit down and read through a pile of evaluation forms. Very often, educators note all the negative comments and ignore or undervalue the compliments they receive. This is typical of human nature and its vulnerability to perceived criticism. However, if the time spent by class participants in completing their evaluation forms is to be respected, then their positive feedback should be as highly valued as their less positive. Evaluation forms are a tool for strengthening teaching and it is as important to acknowledge what has been done well and to build on that as to face up to what has been less successful.

It is common to find in a pile of evaluation forms one or two that are extreme in their comments, either damning the classes from beginning to end or praising everything the educator has done. Those that fall into the first category can be fatal to the educator's self-confidence, and the ones falling into the second are momentarily delightful, but not ultimately very helpful. Whilst neither should be dismissed, it is probably the evaluation forms that provide a balance of praise and criticism that are the most useful. When looking at these, the educator needs to identify themes. If several class members comment that they did not learn much about how to look after their babies or that they considered interventions in labour were not well covered, the educator needs to look at these areas again and, with the help of colleagues, identify some strategies for improving learning opportunities for her clients.

It is very hard not to be demoralized by evaluation forms that seem to contain a lot of criticism. Often, what the educator herself sees as very negative feedback may not appear to be anywhere near as negative to another person. It is therefore important to seek support when dealing with evaluation forms that are short on praise and to check out what clients are really saying with someone else who can look at the feedback more objectively.

After reflecting on the feedback her clients have given her, the educator can then draw up a list of strategies for the future. These need to be couched in very precise terms so that the educator is clear in her own mind about exactly what she needs to do to facilitate learning more effectively in her next course or session; for example:

1. Before the next course, I need to:

- talk to a colleague about ways of incorporating more movement into classes

- read books and articles about adjustment to parenthood

2. During the next course, I need to:

- ensure that I start and finish classes on time

- develop relaxation throughout the course so that people understand how it can be used in labour

- try some new teaching approaches for helping parents understand interventions, especially induction and caesarean section

- ensure that there is much more discussion about looking after babies

FEEDBACK FROM ANOTHER EDUCATOR

Receiving feedback from another colleague is immensely helpful for the educator who wants to evaluate her skills. It is important for the educator to choose someone to observe her classes who is acknowledged to be skilled herself as an educator, who can be trusted to give an honest account of what she has seen, and who will offer *constructive* feedback. Quality feedback not only highlights areas for improvement, but also helps the educator acknowledge what she has done well and build on it. Feedback that is entirely negative does not inspire anyone to do better; it merely demoralizes them. Constructive feedback enables the educator to plan for the future and to feel enthusiastic about working hard to improve her skills. A sensitive observer will understand the nervousness of the person who is being observed and will try hard to set her at ease.

Ideally, the educator needs to meet her observer before the class to tell her a little about the people in the group, the topics that have already been looked at during the course, and what has been planned for the class she is to observe. It is also important to discuss such matters as:

- where the observer will sit

- whether she will participate in activities and discussions

- whether she will take notes during the class

- whether she will be invited to share her own experiences as a mother or as a health professional

- which particular aspects of the class the educator would like to receive feedback about

- when feedback will be given

- whether feedback will be given verbally or in writing, or both

Feedback could be provided in the following areas:

1. the way in which the educator helps group members feel at ease

2. her skill in facilitating discussion

3. her skill in facilitating practical work

4. her ability to give information clearly and concisely

5. her use of language – sensitive? at the appropriate level? reflective of equal opportunities issues?

6. the visual aids she uses – well selected? well displayed?

7. the structure of her class – logical? flexible? balanced between information giving and sharing/discussion/practical work?

8. the way in which she listens to parents and responds to what they are saying

9. the picture she paints of labour and birth

10. her skill in building parents' confidence in their ability to give birth

11. the picture she paints of early parenting

12. her skill in building parents' confidence in their ability to look after their babies

13. the way in which she encourages people to seek information so that they can give informed consent

The observer should offer feedback in the form of a 'sandwich', starting with praise for what the educator did well during her class, proceeding to areas where improvement could be made and discussing how this might be achieved, and finishing by emphasizing again the highlights of the class. Feedback may leave the educator feeling that she has a lot to learn, but she should also have clear ideas about how to move forward and still have lots of enthusiasm.

Conclusion

The following is an extract from feedback given by a skilled observer. It is rich in insight, constructive in its approach, and leaves the person being assessed with a sense of the value of the work in which she is engaged.

> *You used a variety of approaches to help parents learn and to consolidate their learning. Parents had the chance to share their thoughts in the whole group and in small groups. You developed ideas that had been raised in previous classes and stimulated a lively discussion on the role of labour supporters. Role play provided the opportunity for parents to step into the shoes of other people in their social network and to understand more about how a new baby affects relationships within and beyond the family. There was a lot of practical skills work (relaxation, massage, positions for first stage, quick 'shake-out' relaxation) to break up the discussions.*

> *Some parents tended to dominate the discussions and there were three who did not speak at all. It would be helpful for you to consider whether you could use carefully selected small groups to help dominant members listen more and to draw out those who find it hard to contribute but would clearly like to.*

> *Parents felt able to challenge each other's ideas. They did not feel the need to conform and were prepared to explain their position to the rest of the group who accepted it non-judgementally. You listened well throughout the class, reflecting back parents' ideas to enable them to acknowledge and analyse their feelings.*

> *You need to be especially aware of the importance of considering every aspect of labour and the postnatal period from the point of view of the woman in the group who has mobility problems. You also need to ensure that visual aids can be seen clearly by everyone, and to pass round items such as the pelvis and the fetal scalp electrode so that people can learn by handling them.*

> *The agenda for the course had been agreed by yourself and the group members at the start of the course and, when time ran short during this class, you invited them to choose the topics they most wanted to cover. Feedback from the group at the end of the class was very positive with many people commenting on how much they looked forward to meeting each other on Thursday evenings.*

KEY POINTS

1. Evaluation starts with aims and learning outcomes.

2. The body language of group members is a primary source of information about their involvement in the class.

3. Listening to the kind of questions being asked by group members gives the educator clues as to the quality of the learning taking place.

4. **Feedback can be given to the educator, by her clients and by colleagues who observe her classes.**

REFERENCE

Daines J, Daines C and Graham B (1994) *Adult Learning, Adult Teaching.* Nottingham: University of Nottingham, Department of Adult Education.

Appendix 1
Self-Help and Support Groups

There are two useful resources for the childbirth educator when referring clients to self-help and professional groups:

Health Information Service
c/o Help for Health Trust, Highcroft, Romsey Road, Winchester SO22 5DH
Tel: 01962 849100
Helpline: 0800 665544
The helpline provides information about counselling services, self-help groups and NHS services throughout the UK.

MIDIRS: *Directory of Maternity Organisations (1997)*
Published by MIDIRS (Midwives Information and Resource Service)
(see Appendix 2)

Some of the principal support groups relevant to parents are listed below in alphabetical order:

Action on Pre-Eclampsia
31–33 College Road, Harrow, Middlesex HA1 1EJ
Tel: 0181 863 3271
Helpline: 01923 266778

Association for Postnatal Illness (APNI)
25 Jerdan Place, London SW6 1BE
Tel: 0171 386 0868

Caesarean Support Network
55 Cooil Drive, Douglas, Isle of Man IM2 2HF
Tel: 01624 661269

Down's Syndrome Association
155 Mitcham Road, London SW17 9PG
Tel: 0181 682 4001

Disability, Pregnancy and Parenthood International
Fifth Floor, 45 Beech Street, London EC2P 2LX
Tel: 0171 628 2811

Gingerbread (for lone parents)
16/17 Clerkenwell Close, London EC1R 0AA
Tel: 0171 336 8183
Helpline: 0171 336 8184

International Home Birth Movement
The Manor, Standlake, Witney, Oxford OX8 7RH
Tel: 01865 300266 and 01865 300154

Miscarriage Association
c/o Clayton Hospital, Northgate, Wakefield, West Yorkshire WF1 3JS
Tel: 01924 200799

Multiple Births Foundation (MBF)
Queen Charlotte's and Chelsea Hospital, Goldhawk Road, London W6 0XG
Tel: 0181 383 3519

National Childbirth Trust (NCT)
Alexandra House, Oldham Terrace, London W3 6NH
Tel: 0181 992 8637

Parentability (for disabled parents)
Alexandra House, Oldham Terrace, London W3 6NH
Tel: 0181 992 8637

Parent to Parent Information on Adoption Services (PPIAS)
Lower Boddington, Daventry, Northants NN11 6YB
Tel: 01327 26095

SCOPE (for people with cerebral palsy)
12 Park Crescent, London W1N 4EQ
Tel: 0171 636 5020
Helpline: 0800 626 216

Stillbirth and Neonatal Death Society (SANDS)
28 Portland Place, London W1N 4DE
Tel: 0171 436 7940
Helpline: 0171 436 5881

Support Around Termination for Abnormality (SATFA)
73–75 Charlotte Street, London W1P 1LB
Tel: 0171 631 0285
Helpline: 0171 631 0285

Terrence Higgins Trust (services for people affected by HIV)
52–54 Grays Inn Road, London WC1X 8JU
Tel: 0171 831 0330
Helpline: 0171 405 2381

Twins and Multiple Births Association (TAMBA)
PO Box 30, Little Sutton, South Wirral L66 1TH
Tel: 0151 348 0020
Helpline: 01732 868000

APPENDIX 2
Teaching Aids for Childbirth Education Classes

Teaching aids useful for childbirth education classes can be obtained from:

ACE Graphics
PO Box 173, Sevenoaks, Kent TN14 5ZT
Tel: 01959 524622
Catalogue includes books, leaflets, videos, audiocassettes, birth charts, breastfeeding promotional charts, model pelvises, teaching dolls, breast models.

Adam Rouilly Ltd
Crown Quay Lane, Sittingbourne, Kent ME10 3JG
Tel: 01795 471378
Catalogue includes teaching dolls, model pelvises, pregnancy and birth charts.

E & S Products Ltd
A2 Dominion Way, Rustington, West Sussex BN16 3HQ
Tel: 01903 773340
Catalogue includes models of the baby in the womb, pregnancy and birth charts, model pelvises, models of the pelvic floor, teaching dolls.

MIDIRS (Midwives Information and Resource Service)
9 Elmdale Road, Bristol BS8 1SL
Tel: 0117 925 1791
Freephone orderline and enquiry service: 0800 581009
Catalogue includes books, birth charts, videos.

National Childbirth Trust Maternity Sales
239 Shawbridge Street, Glasgow G43 1QN
Tel: 0141 636 0600
Catalogue includes books, leaflets, birth charts, model pelvises, breastfeeding promotion charts, videos, audiocassettes.

Appendix 3
Bibliography of Texts about Childbirth Education

Black TM and Faulkner A (1988) *Ante-Natal Group Skills Training*. Chichester: Wiley.

Brayshaw E and Wright P (1994) *Teaching Physical Skills for the Childbearing Year*. Hale: Books for Midwives Press.

Nichols FH and Humenick SS (1988) *Childbirth Education: Practice, Research and Theory*. London: WB Saunders.

Payne R (1995) *Relaxation Techniques: A Practical Handbook for the Health Care Professional*. New York: Churchill Livingstone.

Priest J and Schott J (1991) *Leading Antenatal Classes: A Practical Guide*. Oxford: Butterworth–Heinemann.

Pugh G, De'Ath E and Smith C (1994) *Confident Parents, Confident Children: Policy and Practice in Parent Education and Support*. London: National Children's Bureau.

Robertson A (1993) *Preparing for Birth: Background Notes for Prenatal Classes*, 2nd edn. Camperdown, NSW: ACE Graphics.

Robertson A (1994) *Empowering Women – Teaching Active Birth in the '90s*. Camperdown, NSW. Ace Graphics.

Wilberg GM (1992) *Preparing for Birth and Parenthood*. Oxford.

Wilson P (1990) *Antenatal Teaching*. London: Faber

Index

Page numbers in bold type refer to illustrations.

ANTENATAL EDUCATION: A DYNAMIC APPROACH